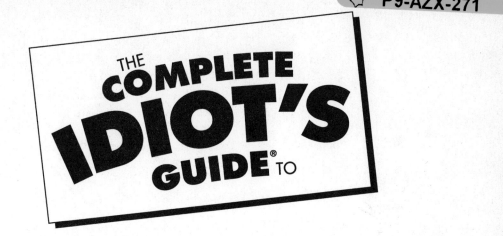

THE COMPLETE IDIOT'S GUIDE® TO

Flour-Free Eating

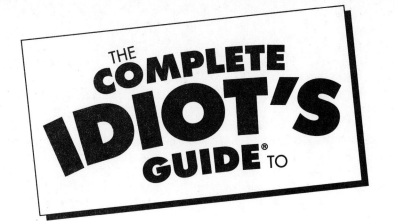

Flour-Free Eating

*by Keith Wayne Berkowitz, M.D.,
and Shelly Vaughan James*

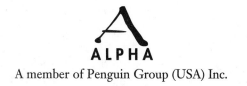

ALPHA

A member of Penguin Group (USA) Inc.

ALPHA BOOKS

Published by the Penguin Group

Penguin Group (USA) Inc., 375 Hudson Street, New York, New York 10014, USA

Penguin Group (Canada), 90 Eglinton Avenue East, Suite 700, Toronto, Ontario M4P 2Y3, Canada (a division of Pearson Penguin Canada Inc.)

Penguin Books Ltd., 80 Strand, London WC2R 0RL, England

Penguin Ireland, 25 St. Stephen's Green, Dublin 2, Ireland (a division of Penguin Books Ltd.)

Penguin Group (Australia), 250 Camberwell Road, Camberwell, Victoria 3124, Australia (a division of Pearson Australia Group Pty. Ltd.)

Penguin Books India Pvt. Ltd., 11 Community Centre, Panchsheel Park, New Delhi—110 017, India

Penguin Group (NZ), 67 Apollo Drive, Rosedale, North Shore, Auckland 1311, New Zealand (a division of Pearson New Zealand Ltd.)

Penguin Books (South Africa) (Pty.) Ltd., 24 Sturdee Avenue, Rosebank, Johannesburg 2196, South Africa

Penguin Books Ltd., Registered Offices: 80 Strand, London WC2R 0RL, England

International Standard Book Number: 978-1-61564-027-0
Library of Congress Catalog Card Number: 2009941621

12 11 10   8 7 6 5 4 3 2 1

Interpretation of the printing code: The rightmost number of the first series of numbers is the year of the book's printing; the rightmost number of the second series of numbers is the number of the book's printing. For example, a printing code of 10-1 shows that the first printing occurred in 2010.

Printed in the United States of America

Note: This publication contains the opinions and ideas of its authors. It is intended to provide helpful and informative material on the subject matter covered. It is sold with the understanding that the authors and publisher are not engaged in rendering professional services in the book. If the reader requires personal assistance or advice, a competent professional should be consulted.

The authors and publisher specifically disclaim any responsibility for any liability, loss, or risk, personal or otherwise, which is incurred as a consequence, directly or indirectly, of the use and application of any of the contents of this book.

Most Alpha books are available at special quantity discounts for bulk purchases for sales promotions, premiums, fundraising, or educational use. Special books, or book excerpts, can also be created to fit specific needs.

For details, write: Special Markets, Alpha Books, 375 Hudson Street, New York, NY 10014.

Publisher: *Marie Butler-Knight*
Associate Publisher: *Mike Sanders*
Senior Managing Editor: *Billy Fields*
Acquisitions Editor: *Tom Stevens*
Development Editor: *Ginny Bess Munroe*
Production Editor: *Kayla Dugger*

Copy Editor: *Tricia Liebig*
Cover Designer: *Bill Thomas*
Book Designer: *Trina Wurst*
Indexer: *Julie Bess*
Layout: *Ayanna Lacey*
Proofreader: *John Etchison*

To Valerie, my daily inspiration. —Keith
For Lewis, who, in the end, knew I was going somewhere. —Shelly

Contents at a Glance

Contents

Introduction

You may have picked up this cookbook in search of better nutrition and recipes that fit your dietary needs. Naturally, we've included mouthwatering recipes, all of them flour-free. We share foods we think you'll love, as well as dishes that will intrigue your taste buds with new flavors and combinations.

Beyond the appetizing recipes, we've shared valuable information on how flour affects your health. Equipped with essential information, you can take charge of your diet, helping to avert potential health problems, such as obesity, high blood pressure, heart disease, cancers, type 2 diabetes, and more.

With good information and flour-free recipes, you can cook and eat, being mindful of the health advantages for your body. Our hope is that you'll take away what you've learned and put into practice the measures and methods you need to live a more healthful life without feeling restricted in your ability to put together a delicious, nourishing meal.

Here's to your good health!

How This Book Is Organized

This book is divided into five parts:

Part 1, "Achieve Flour Freedom," presents indispensible information on flour, carbohydrates, insulin, and more that you need to cook and eat flour-free foods. You'll learn how to read nutrition labels and find flours in your diet. We introduce you to flour alternatives and ways to enjoy meals without using flour products.

Part 2, "Better Breakfasts, Brunches, and Breads," features recipes you'll enjoy as sunrise selections, as well as quick breads and muffins that can start your day or satisfy your hunger pangs any time of day.

Part 3, "Lunches and Lighter Fare," provides midday ideas and smart snacks. You'll find plenty of recipes for sandwiches, soups, stews, salads, appetizers, and tasty tidbits.

Part 4, "Mealtime Makeovers," satisfies your need for entrées and side dishes from simple to spectacular. Whether you're hungry for beef, pork, chicken, turkey, fish, seafood, meatless meals, or great go-withs, you'll find the recipe here.

Part 5, "Dilemma-Solving Desserts," pleases your sweet tooth with recipes for delectable indulgences. Treat yourself to cakes, cookies, brownies, pies, puddings, and more scrumptious sweets.

Flour-Free Flourishes

You'll come across many sidebars throughout this book that offer you a little something extra. Here's what to look for:

For Good Measure

Facts shared in these boxes impart extraneous tidbits you can use to impress your friends—and maybe win a trivia game.

Words to Digest

These boxes extend definitions for helpful vocabulary for eating and cooking flour-free.

Starch Guard

Keep an eye out for these boxes. While some may contain info about hidden flours or starches, others may present serious warnings to avoid possible problems.

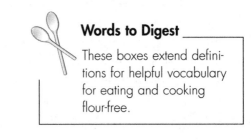

No-Flour Power

Filled with all kinds of ways to make something easier, these boxes are fantastically valuable. You'll find information to help you eat more healthfully and work more efficiently in the kitchen.

Acknowledgments

While only two names are credited on the cover of this book, we are all too aware of the contributions afforded by many others who made this book possible.

Keith would like to thank his wife, Valerie, for her guidance and wisdom on this path to better health and wellness. To his three children and the rest of the Berkowitz family: "It is your daily inspiration and never-wavering support that have been critical to keeping me on course." He also wants to thank Beata Moniuszko and Binni Ipcar, whose dedication and passion have been essential to the success of his medical practice, The Center for Balanced Health.

Shelly would like to thank her husband, Bob, and daughter, Bethany, for their patience and understanding during her long work hours. She would also like to thank all the taste testers: Garry and Mary Ellen Goldsmith, Michael Goldsmith, Rick Goldsmith, Ron and Sandy Horky, Bob James, David and Julie James, Tyler James, Katelyn James, Bob and MaryLou James, Phyllis McNell, Paul and Patty Ondrick,

Kathy Sechrest, Matt Sechrest, Luetta Trigg, Scott and Kari Werkhoven, Kadyn Werkhoven, Bob and Kaylene Wilson, and Jeff Wilson. It's a tasty job, but somebody has to do it!

We extend a big thank you to Tom Stevens, our acquisitions editor at Alpha, whose guidance helped shape this book into the best it could be. We thank our development editor, Ginny Munroe, production editor, Kayla Dugger, and copy editor, Tricia Liebig, for pruning our manuscript for accuracy and readability. We would also like to thank Marilyn Allen of the Allen O'Shea Literary Agency, whose confidence in our abilities advances us on our career paths.

Special Thanks to the Technical Reviewer

The Complete Idiot's Guide to Flour-Free Eating was reviewed by an expert who double-checked the accuracy of what you'll learn here, to help us ensure that this book gives you everything you need to know about cooking and eating flour-free. Special thanks are extended to Jennifer Anderson.

Trademarks

All terms mentioned in this book that are known to be or are suspected of being trademarks or service marks have been appropriately capitalized. Alpha Books and Penguin Group (USA) Inc. cannot attest to the accuracy of this information. Use of a term in this book should not be regarded as affecting the validity of any trademark or service mark.

Part 1

Achieve Flour Freedom

Refined white and wheat flours offer little in the way of nutrients, vitamins, and minerals. Plus, these overly processed ingredients are made up of simple glucose units that cause an increase in blood sugar levels, and thereby an increase in insulin secretion. Increased insulin can be linked to a number of health issues, including obesity, high blood pressure, heart disease, cancers, type 2 diabetes, and others.

Take heart! You can easily achieve flour-free eating. A quick kitchen makeover to incorporate flour substitutes, better nutrition information, and plenty of delectable recipes will have you eating flour-free for your health.

Chapter 1

The Scoop on Flour and Carbs

In This Chapter

- ◆ The problem with flour
- ◆ Simple carbohydrates of common sugars
- ◆ More slowly digested complex carbohydrates
- ◆ The benefits of soluble and insoluble fiber

Everyone's trying to limit their sugar intake. The epidemic increase in diabetes and obesity has made us more selective about the foods we eat. As a result, sugar-free foods are starting to dominate the marketplace. Unfortunately, sugar is only half the problem. The other half is starch-based carbohydrates which like sugar can have a negative impact on your blood glucose level.

An excellent way to decrease your carbohydrate intake and limit your sugar consumption is through flour-free eating. In this chapter, you learn that not all carbohydrates are created equal. Simple carbohydrates and starch-based complex carbohydrates have a much greater impact on your blood glucose level than fiber-rich complex carbohydrates.

Eating Flour-Free

The other half of the problem is white and wheat flour. Like sugar, both white and wheat flours are refined products that offer very little in terms of vitamins, nutrients, and/or minerals. Although sugar is a simple carbohydrate and white and wheat flours are complex carbohydrates, both are made up of simple glucose units. Therefore, both white and wheat flours cause an increase in your blood glucose level. An elevated blood glucose level stimulates the pancreas to secrete *insulin*.

Words to Digest

Insulin, a hormone secreted by the pancreas, is responsible for helping tissues utilize glucose and amino acids.

As the body is exposed to more and more insulin, insulin resistance develops. Insulin resistance occurs when the pancreas has to secrete great amounts of insulin in order to help tissues utilize glucose and amino acids. This creates a vicious cycle, which in the long run leads to "burnout"—the pancreas is no longer able to meet the demand for insulin, resulting in type 2 diabetes.

An elevated insulin level is also the underlying factor in other health problems, including obesity, heart disease, high blood pressure, osteoporosis, and cancer. The key to preventing these health conditions is keeping blood glucose levels stable and insulin levels low.

Through reading this book, you learn how different macronutrients, including protein, fat, and carbohydrates, play a role in this process. Carbohydrates, including flour, have a greater impact on blood glucose levels than protein and fat.

The alternative is flour-free eating. You can prepare nutritionally rich and delicious recipes without using flour. These natural ingredients are better sources of fiber, protein, and fat, making them great flour substitutes:

- Almond meal
- Ground coconut
- Chia seeds
- Konjac noodles
- Amaranth
- Quinoa
- Stone-ground cornmeal

- ◆ Brown rice meal
- ◆ Flaxseed meal
- ◆ Ground fava beans
- ◆ Ground hazelnuts
- ◆ Ground garbanzo beans
- ◆ Sorghum
- ◆ Steel-cut oats
- ◆ Soba noodles

Using these ingredients as a flour-free foundation, your palate will be so satisfied you won't miss the flour.

Comprehending Carbohydrates

Carbohydrates, the body's main energy source, are composed of carbon, hydrogen, and oxygen atoms that form a sugar unit. One or more of these sugar units bond to make a carbohydrate. When digested, carbohydrates are transported to the liver and used as energy by any body tissue or stored in the liver or muscles as glycogen. When full, excess carbohydrates are stored in fat cells.

Not all carbohydrates are created equal. Traditionally, carbohydrates are divided into categories: simple or complex. Although both groups provide us with energy equal to 4 calories per gram, they differ in chemical structure.

Simple Carbohydrates

Simple carbohydrates, better known as simple sugars, are composed of either a single-sugar unit, monosaccharide, or a two-sugar unit, disaccharide. Examples of monosaccharides include glucose (found in candy), fructose (found in fruit and honey), and galactose (found in milk sugar).

Glucose, also known as dextrose, is the most common form of sugar and the end energy product. Both fructose and galactose are converted to glucose so the body can better utilize them. These simple sugars tend to contain few essential vitamins and minerals and have a detrimental impact on blood glucose levels. Following is a list of monosaccharides and their corresponding food ingredients.

Monosaccharides	Food Ingredients
Glucose	Corn syrup
Fructose	Fruit sugar
	High-fructose corn syrup
Fructose and Glucose	Honey

For Good Measure

Stevia, a sugar substitute derived from the Stevia or Sugarleaf plant, is 300 times sweeter than sugar. With its slower onset and longer duration of action than sugar, the substitute is showing up in diet soft drinks, low-carb foods, and low-sugar options. Select carefully, as some extracts have a bitter or licorice-like after-taste at high concentrations.

Disaccharides, popularly described as double sugars, are composed of two single-sugar units, or monosaccharides, bound together. The three most common disaccharides are sucrose, maltose, and lactose. Sucrose and maltose are much easier for the body to digest than lactose and may have a greater impact on blood glucose levels. Following is a list of disaccharides and their corresponding food ingredients.

Disaccharides	Food Ingredients
Sucrose	Beet or cane sugar
(Fructose and Glucose)	Brown sugar
	Maple syrup
	Powdered sugar
	White sugar
Maltose	Malt sugar
(Glucose and Glucose)	
Lactose	Milk sugar
(Glucose and Galactose)	

No-Flour Power _____

Agave syrup or nectar is a sugar substitute that comes from the Blue Agave or Tequila Agave plant in Mexico. The syrup is a disaccharide, primarily fructose and glucose. Agave syrup's advantage is that it is sweeter than honey and has a smaller impact on blood glucose levels than most natural sweeteners.

Complex Carbohydrates

Complex carbohydrates, known as polysaccharides, are composed of multiple sugar units in long chains, or polymers. Unlike simple carbohydrates, complex carbohydrates take longer to digest. They also contain fiber, vitamins, and minerals. Examples of complex carbohydrates include vegetables, cereals, breads, legumes, and pasta. The three most important complex carbohydrates are starch, glycogen, and dietary fiber:

♦ *Starch* is the most common type of complex carbohydrate and consists of multiple strands of glucose units linked together. The main form of energy storage for plants, it can be broken down by human enzymes into individual glucose units. Known as the digestible polysaccharide, starch is digested at the beginning of the large intestine. Starches include pasta and breads.

♦ *Glycogen* is another complex carbohydrate and, like starch, consists of strands of glucose units bonded together. Unlike starch, glycogen is the main source of energy in humans and animals. Glycogen's advantage is that it is more effectively utilized as glucose by the body than starch.

♦ *Dietary fiber* is a third complex carbohydrate consisting of multiple glucose units bound together. Unlike starch and glycogen, dietary fiber is not digested at the beginning of the large intestine and is not a significant source of energy. Dietary fiber plays an important role in regulating blood cholesterol levels and blood glucose levels and removing toxic waste from the digestive tract.

Dietary fiber is found in two types. Dietary fiber is either soluble or insoluble, depending on its ability to hold water.

For Good Measure _____

According to the American Dietetic Association, the average American consumes only 14 to 15 grams of fiber a day, far less than the recommended 25 to 35 grams a day. The breakdown of fiber in an average American diet is 75 percent insoluble and 25 percent soluble.

Soluble fiber is differentiated by its ability to form a gel when mixed with fatty acids or liquids. This mixture slows stomach emptying so that sugar is released—and subsequently absorbed—more slowly and therefore improves blood glucose levels. Soluble fiber also reduces low-density lipoproteins (LDL or bad cholesterol). Foods high in soluble fiber include the following:

- Oats and oat bran

- Dried beans and peas

- Nuts

- Barley

- Oranges, pears, and apples

- Carrots

- Psyllium husks

Insoluble fiber doesn't mix with liquid and passes through the large intestines intact. Insoluble fiber keeps the bowels regular and removes toxic waste from the body. Food sources of insoluble fiber include the following:

- Green beans and dark green, leafy vegetables

- Fruit skins

- Root vegetable skins

- Whole-wheat–based foods

- Wheat bran

- Corn bran

- Seeds and nuts

Many foods contain both insoluble and soluble fiber, such as oats, oat bran, psyllium husks, and flaxseed.

For Good Measure _____

Functional fibers are a new category of fibers now available. Either isolated from natural sources and/or synthetic nondigestible carbohydrates, the two most common types of functional fibers are inulin and fructoligosaccharides (FOS). Inulin is extracted from chicory root, while FOS is derived from beet or cane sugar. These fibers are often used as an ingredient in yogurt and baked goods.

The Least You Need to Know

- White and wheat flours, being refined products, provide few vitamins, nutrients, and minerals.

- White and wheat flours increase blood glucose levels, stimulating the secretion of insulin by the pancreas.

- Carbohydrates are the body's primary source of energy, but not all carbohydrates are treated the same by your body.

- Simple carbohydrates negatively affect blood glucose levels.

- Complex carbohydrates are slowly digested, gradually releasing sugars while supplying fiber, vitamins, and minerals.

Dangerous Course of Insulin

In This Chapter

◆ Insulin's role in the body

◆ Starch and sugar's impact on insulin

◆ How increased insulin affects your health

A hormone secreted by the pancreas in correlation with blood glucose levels, insulin plays a major part in your body's functioning and overall health. Spikes in blood sugar—increased by both sugars and starches—can be detrimental. Stabilizing blood glucose levels is instrumental for your body's best performance. Following a flour-free diet can help you better accomplish this goal.

The focus of this chapter is on insulin and its impact on the body, including metabolism. Elevated blood glucose levels lead to elevated insulin levels. Over time, these elevated insulin levels become dangerous to your health by increasing your risk of high blood pressure, heart disease, obesity, type 2 diabetes, osteoporosis, and thyroid dysfunction.

The Function of Insulin

Secreted by the pancreas, insulin helps tissues utilize glucose and amino acids. In this role, insulin keeps both metabolism and blood glucose levels stable.

Secretion of insulin is dependent on the concentration of glucose in the bloodstream. The greater the blood glucose level, the greater the secretion of insulin by the pancreas. Insulin lowers the blood glucose level by storing the glucose as glycogen in the liver and in muscle tissue. When these stores are full, any excess is converted to fat and stored in *adipose tissue*. This mechanism helps the body store energy for later use when the body has no food available.

Words to Digest

Adipose tissue is a type of connective tissue that stores cellular fat. The most common types in humans are subcutaneous and visceral fat. Subcutaneous is the type beneath the skin while visceral is the type that surrounds internal organs. An elevated amount of visceral fat is linked to an increased risk of heart disease.

Impact on Metabolism

As the body is exposed to increased amounts of glucose, the pancreas has to respond by secreting more insulin. With increased sugar consumption, the problem is the simultaneous increase in insulin production. Cells and tissues exposed to greater loads of insulin become more resistant to the insulin, leading to an even greater production of insulin by the pancreas. Unfortunately, not all cells and tissues become equally resistant. The liver and muscle tissues develop resistance much sooner than do fat cells. The body then stores more and more glucose as glycogen in fat cells, resulting in waistline expansion.

For Good Measure

In the last 20 years, the average person has increased annual sugar consumption from 26 pounds to 135 pounds—equivalent to 20 teaspoons of sugar per person per day.

The pancreas in some individuals increases production by as much as 10 times to keep up with the increased demand. The body doesn't have an unlimited supply of insulin, so the pancreas is unable to keep up with an increased demand forever. The body is placed in a catch-22 of decreased insulin production at the same time it is faced with an increased insulin resistance. Higher blood glucose levels and the development of type 2 diabetes results.

Bearing on Blood Sugar

With an understanding of the relationship between blood glucose and insulin, the goal is to learn how to stabilize blood glucose levels. Stabilizing blood glucose levels lowers insulin secretion and decreases insulin resistance. By lowering sugar consumption, you avoid "the blood sugar roller coaster."

This perpetual cycle has led to dramatic increases in sugar consumption. In 1983, sugar consumption represented 11 percent of daily caloric intake. Today, it's 15 percent, an increase of 30 percent in only 25 years. The U.S. Department of Agriculture recommends a daily intake of sugar limited to 8 percent of the daily caloric intake, or 10 teaspoons per person per day—a 50 percent decrease from current levels.

Symptoms of Unstable Blood Glucose

Individuals who develop insulin resistance often develop the following symptoms after a high sugar or starch meal:

♦ **Hunger.** After a meal full of carbohydrates, blood sugar goes up quickly, and then falls just as quickly, causing individuals to feel as though they've not eaten.

♦ **Fatigue/sleepiness.** Increased insulin resistance causes blood glucose to fall, which leaves individuals without energy and exhausted.

♦ **"Brain fog."** Low blood glucose makes it difficult to concentrate and focus on everyday tasks.

♦ **Gas and bloating.** Most gas is produced because the large intestine cannot handle the carbohydrate load.

♦ **Irritability.** Mood is affected by blood glucose levels. The brain is the largest consumer of glucose in the body and the most sensitive to changes in blood glucose levels.

Insulin's Effect on Health

If we had to pick a medical villain today, insulin would be fingered. Research has linked high insulin levels as a causative factor in numerous medical conditions.

Obesity

Increased insulin levels facilitate the conversion of excess glucose to glycogen, which is stored as fat after energy demands are met and liver and muscle stores are full. To compound this problem, insulin then takes carbohydrates supplied in the diet and utilizes them for energy while leaving fat stores intact.

Diet changes, specifically an increase in refined carbohydrates, has led to the ever-increasing American waistline. According to the Centers for Disease Control (CDC), two thirds of Americans are overweight, of whom half are also obese. This is defined using the body mass index (BMI), a relative percentage of fat and muscle mass in the body calculated using a person's height and weight. Individuals with a BMI between 25 and 29.9 are considered overweight, while those above 30 are considered obese.

High Blood Pressure

Elevated insulin levels can lead to high blood pressure because of insulin's effect on two essential electrolytes: *magnesium* and *sodium*.

Words to Digest

Magnesium is an essential nutrient required for all energy-producing reactions that take place in the cells and muscles, including the ability to relax.

Sodium is an essential nutrient that is required for the normal functioning of muscle and nerve cells. Excess amounts of sodium can lead to water retention.

Elevated insulin levels cause the body to excrete magnesium. When magnesium levels are low, blood vessels constrict, causing blood pressure to rise. A long-standing elevated blood pressure increases the risk of heart disease, stroke, and kidney failure.

When insulin levels are elevated, sodium retention is also elevated. This causes fluid retention, which increases blood pressure.

Heart Disease

Insulin plays a key role in the development of heart disease. As previously described, excess insulin makes blood vessels lose their ability to relax. When arteries become less elastic, stress causes cracks and fractures within the arterial walls. Cholesterol builds up to seal these weaknesses, causing the build-up of plaque within the arteries.

Plaque is made from substances that circulate in the bloodstream that include calcium, fat, cholesterol, cellular waste products, and fibrin. Fibrin is a protein that plays a role in blood clotting. This plaque decreases bloodflow to the heart and increases the risk of a heart attack.

Insulin can also cause the liver to produce increased levels of triglycerides. Individuals, especially women, with an elevated triglyceride level are at increased risk for heart disease.

Symptoms of metabolic syndrome include:

♦ **Abdominal obesity**—Excessive fat tissue around the abdomen.

♦ **Cholesterol disorders**—High triglycerides, low HDL (good) cholesterol, and high LDL (bad) cholesterol.

♦ **High blood pressure.**

♦ **Insulin resistance or increased glucose level.**

♦ **High C-reactive protein**—A marker of inflammation.

♦ **Increased fibrinogen**—A marker of increased risk of blood clotting or thrombosis.

Type 2 Diabetes

Prolonged elevated insulin levels cause cells and tissues to become more resistant to insulin. As mentioned before, this leads to a greater production of insulin by the pancreas to meet demand. Eventually, insulin production falls short, and blood glucose levels rise, causing type 2 diabetes. Type 2 diabetes is defined as a fasting blood glucose level of 125 or a random blood glucose level above 200.

Osteoporosis

Insulin acts as the "master hormone," controlling the hormones that affect the building of bones and muscle growth. This process is reduced in the setting of insulin resistance, and the production of the growth hormone, testosterone, and progesterone is reduced. The end result is a decrease in bone building and an increase in calcium excretion. This leads to osteoporosis, a thinning of the bone and the loss of bone density. Osteoporosis occurs most often in postmenopausal women and places individuals at an increased risk of falling and developing fractures.

Thyroid

The thyroid gland produces the hormone T4, which is transported to the liver for conversion to T3. For tissues to utilize the thyroid hormone, this conversion to the active form, T3, must occur. When the liver becomes insulin-resistant, it can no longer complete this conversion; tissues and other organs aren't supplied with the needed thyroid hormone.

Cancer

Insulin is an important regulatory hormone for cell growth. This is true for both normal and cancer cells. High insulin levels are now shown to have the strongest correlation for the development of colon, prostate, and breast cancers.

A study in *The Journal of the National Cancer Institute* showed that men with higher insulin are at increased risk for prostate cancer. Women with high insulin levels are eight times (32 percent versus 4 percent) more likely to die within seven years after diagnosis of breast cancer, according to a study of 535 women at the University of Toronto School of Medicine.

Starch and Sugar Give Rise to Insulin

A common mistake is to forget that starches raise blood glucose levels in the same way as sugars. A sugar-free food can still increase blood glucose levels and, in turn, elevate insulin. A food product with 3 grams of sugar has less impact on blood glucose level than a sugar-free product with 20 grams of starch.

Remember, sugar and starch both come from a single glucose unit. The main difference between starch and sugar is the number of units linked together. Sugar is only one or two simple-sugar units, while starch is a multiple-bonded, simple-sugar unit. Sugar, a simple carbohydrate, is digested and utilized as glucose more quickly than starch, a complex carbohydrate. Still, both sugar and starch raise blood glucose levels—sugar just gets there faster.

The Least You Need to Know

- Insulin secretion is in direct correlation to blood glucose levels and is most healthful when stabilized.
- Excess glucose is stored as glycogen in fat cells, resulting in a larger waistline.

◆ Increased insulin can be linked to a number of health problems, including obesity, high blood pressure, heart disease, type 2 diabetes, osteoporosis, and cancer.

◆ Starches raise blood glucose levels in the same way as sugars.

Getting Ingrained in Nutrition

In This Chapter

- ◆ Nutritional components of the foods you eat
- ◆ Your body's use of calories
- ◆ "Good" fats and "bad" fats and their differences

Before you begin the journey of a flour-free lifestyle, learning basic nutritional principles can provide guidance. You will learn about two critical macronutrients: fat and protein. Fat has been called public enemy number one in the fight against obesity. Unfortunately, it is not this simple, for not all fats are created equal. In addition, you will learn that sodium, often vilified by many nutritional experts, plays an essential role within the human body.

Calories

Any food decision must start with the *calorie*. Calories are the road map to determine how much energy is in the food we eat. For example, a 200-calorie food will provide the body with 200 calories of energy. The number of calories in a single food is determined by evaluating the macronutrients that help our bodies function effectively—our three old friends: fat, protein, and carbohydrates. Carbohydrates were covered in Chapter 1.

Words to Digest

The **calorie** is defined as the amount of energy required to raise the temperature of 1 gram of water 1°C. This basic unit of energy is often called the calorie (with a lowercase c). One thousand calories are known as 1 kilocalorie—the amount of energy contained in food and released upon digestion by the human body. Unfortunately, this terminology can be confusing because on a nutrition label kilocalories are labeled as Calories. One Calorie (with a capital C) is equivalent to 1,000 calories.

Fat is the most energy efficient of the macronutrients, providing 9 calories of energy per gram. Protein and carbohydrate both provide only 4 calories of energy per gram.

All macronutrients provide calories of energy except dietary fiber. Dietary fiber is a form of carbohydrate that is not digested by the body. It neither provides calorie energy nor counts toward the caloric value of a food.

Fat

Fat, also known as fatty acid, plays an essential role in keeping our bodies functioning efficiently. After digestion, most fats are carried into the bloodstream and stored until they're processed by our cells to be used directly for energy. When called upon by the body, they're either broken down by the energy plant of each individual cell or by the liver through a process of *ketosis*.

Words to Digest

Ketosis occurs when the body goes through a prolonged period of starvation that produces dangerously high levels of ketones. Or it occurs when the body ingests large quantities of fat in the absence of carbohydrates, producing a minimal increase of ketones. In this case, ketones substitute for glucose as an energy source.

Contrary to popular belief, fat is an important nutrient and plays a key role in ensuring the body stays healthy by …

- Maintaining cell membrane structure.

- Aiding normal brain development in children.

- Transporting the fat-soluble vitamins A, D, E, and K.

- Helping the body manufacture antibodies to fight disease.

- Acting as a cushion to protect our internal organs.

- Supplying critical nutrients, such as essential fatty acids.

- Providing a long-term energy reserve.

Most people are surprised to learn that fat plays an important role in maintaining a healthy body. Not all fats are created equal, of course, as fats can be good or bad. For our discussion, fats can be classified into four categories: saturated, monounsaturated, polyunsaturated, and trans fats.

Saturated Fats

Again and again, we're told to consume less saturated fat because it raises cholesterol and increases our risk of heart disease. This statement oversimplifies the role of saturated fats.

Saturated fat is a fatty acid produced from triglycerides. Unlike the other fats, it's fully saturated with hydrogen atoms and therefore becomes solid at room temperature. Saturated fats are further classified as long-, medium-, or short-chain triglycerides. The majority of fat-based foods we eat are long-chain triglycerides.

For Good Measure _____

Medium-chain triglycerides (MCTs), unlike the other two saturated fats, are digested quickly by the body. Most fats are broken down in the intestines and then transported by the blood for later usage. MCTs are absorbed intact and can be used immediately for energy, similar to carbohydrates. Research suggests that MCTs may help promote weight-loss and improve athletic performance. The best sources of MCTs are palm oil and coconut oil.

Saturated fats are found in numerous food products, including the following:

Short-Chain Triglycerides

- Cow's milk

- Sheep's milk

- Goat's milk

Medium-Chain Triglycerides

- Coconut oil

- Palm kernel oil

- Butter

Long-Chain Triglycerides

- Butter

- Red meat

- Chocolate

- Solid shortenings

- Eggs

Monounsaturated Fats

Monounsaturated fats differ from saturated fats in that they are simple fatty acids. Monounsaturated fats aren't completely saturated with hydrogen atoms and are typically liquid at room temperature, only solidifying when cooled. Most nutritional experts consider monounsaturated fats the "good" or "healthy" fats because they lower bad (LDL) cholesterol and contain excellent amounts of vitamin E.

Monounsaturated fat is found in numerous food products, including these:

- Avocados

- Olive oil and olives

- Almonds, pecans, peanuts, and cashews

- Peanut, cashew, and almond butters

- Sesame seeds

- Canola oil

Polyunsaturated Fats

Polyunsaturated fats are complex fatty acids and are even less saturated with hydrogen atoms. They are liquid at room temperature and when cooled. Two essential polyunsaturated fats are omega 3s and omega 6s.

Omega 3s reduce serum (total) *cholesterol* levels, decrease inflammation, and prevent clogging of the arteries. Omega 6s reduce pain, decrease premenstrual symptoms, and prevent neuropathy.

Polyunsaturated fat is found in numerous food products, including the following:

- Corn, cottonseed, safflower, sunflower, and soybean oils
- Walnuts
- Pumpkin and sunflower seeds
- Mayonnaise made with soybean oil
- Salad dressings made with soybean oil

Foods high in omega 3s include these:

- Herring, mackerel, rainbow trout, salmon, and sardines (including oils)
- Green leafy vegetables
- Flaxseed
- Hemp
- Walnuts
- Tofu

Foods high in omega 6s include these:

- Flaxseed and flaxseed oil
- Hemp seeds and hempseed oil
- Pumpkin seeds
- Walnut oil
- Pine nuts and pistachios
- Olives and olive oil

Words to Digest

Cholesterol is a form of fat called a sterol found in animal and plant tissue. In humans, the liver manufactures cholesterol, and it's absorbed from food in the intestine. Cholesterol is a major component of blood plasma and cell membranes and is important for brain and nerve function. It is also a precursor in the production of vitamin D2, estrogen, testosterone, and cortisol.

Whether dietary cholesterol actually increases serum cholesterol is unclear. Studies of eggs, which are high in cholesterol, have suggested that eating eggs does not increase the risk for coronary heart disease or increase serum cholesterol levels. Foods high in cholesterol include egg yolks, liver, high-fat meats and poultry skin, and high-fat dairy products.

Trans Fats

Trans fats are created when a liquid oil, typically vegetable, is turned into a solid. The process is called *hydrogenation*. The double bonds of monounsaturated fats or poly-unsaturated fats are artificially broken so hydrogen atoms can be added. This process creates a saturated fat that is now solid at room temperature.

Trans fats raise bad (LDL) cholesterol and lower good (HDL) cholesterol, increasing the risk for heart disease, stroke, and type 2 diabetes. Trans fats often appear as hydrogenated or partially hydrogenated oils on nutrition labels.

Trans fats are found in numerous food products, including:

♦ Margarine

♦ Vegetable shortenings

♦ Fast food items (e.g., french fries)

♦ Processed snacks and baked goods

Protein

Protein is a key component in bones, muscles, cartilage, skin, blood, enzymes, and hormones. Considered the human body's "building block," protein is composed of chains of amino acids. Twenty amino acids make up these building blocks, and they fall into two categories: *essential amino acids* and *nonessential amino acids*.

> **Words to Digest** _____
>
> **Essential amino acids** are not produced by the body and need to be supplied in the daily diet. Excellent sources of all nine essential amino acids include eggs, poultry, milk, and quinoa.
>
> **Nonessential amino acids** are produced by the body utilizing raw materials supplied by food. Excellent sources are foods high in protein, including red meat, chicken, turkey, tuna, salmon, eggs, cheese, almonds, peanuts and peanut butter, and yogurt.

During digestion, protein is broken down into amino acids and either used for the body's biological requirements or stored as glycogen or fat. If the body is deficient in carbohydrates or fat, protein is utilized as an energy source. Through a process called gluconeogenesis, protein is converted into glucose by liver and kidney cells.

Foods high in protein include the following:

- Meat
- Poultry
- Eggs
- Cheese
- Legumes
- Fish

Sodium

Americans have increased their sodium consumption from processed foods and restaurant meals. According to the *Journal of the American Medical Association,* 77 percent of our sodium intake comes from these sources. Sodium is generally present in small quantities in natural foods, but excessive consumption of sodium is thought to increase the risk of hypertension and cardiovascular disease.

As sodium is essential to human life, you don't want to eliminate it completely. Sodium is a critical component to all bodily fluids, including blood and sweat. It helps manage internal fluid balance and prevent dehydration. Sodium also plays a role in the following:

- Nerve and brain functioning

- Muscle contraction

- Preventing heat exhaustion

- Preventing sunstroke

- Glucose absorption

- Acid-base balance

- Proper heart function

Food manufacturers must follow guidelines set by the U.S. Food and Drug Administration (FDA) when labeling the sodium content of their products. As always, you need to read the nutrition facts boxes for exact information, but familiarity with sodium-related labeling terms can help you make more healthful choices.

FDA Sodium Labeling Guidelines

Labeling Term	Indication
Sodium-free	Less than 5 mg sodium per serving
Very low-sodium	Up to 35 mg sodium per serving
Low-sodium	No more than 140 mg sodium per serving
Reduced-sodium	Typical sodium content is reduced by 25 percent
Unsalted, no-salt-added, or without added salt	Natural sodium content is not increased during processing

The Least You Need to Know

- Calories reflect the amount of energy a food supplies.

- Fats are necessary to maintain health, but monounsaturated and polyunsaturated fats are better choices.

- Your diet must supply essential amino acids for the composition of protein, the "building block" of the body.

- Sodium is essential for fluid balance in the body, but many Americans consume excessive amounts.

Chapter 4

Putting It All Together

In This Chapter

- ◆ Avoiding unhealthy ingredients found in processed foods
- ◆ Deciphering the serving size of packaged foods
- ◆ Deciding which foods meet your nutritional needs

Knowing that starch and other complex carbohydrates raise blood glucose levels, you can now make better food choices. With flour-free eating, white and wheat flours are replaced with natural, more nutritionally rich alternatives. This foundation for a more balanced diet can reduce the impact on blood glucose levels. In this chapter, you will learn how to better interpret the nutritional information contained within a food label.

Interpreting the Ingredients List

With the introduction of more complex ingredients by food manufacturers, food labels are becoming increasingly more difficult to understand. An educated consumer practically needs a degree in biochemistry and food science to comprehend and place in perspective the complex chemicals used in foods.

Before buying packaged foods, first carefully review all the ingredients listed on the labels. The ingredients list starts with the ingredient used in the largest quantity and ends with the ingredient used in the smallest quantity.

The key to healthy eating is choosing clean, nutrient-rich, real foods. Ingredients to avoid include artificial colors, refined sugars like evaporated cane juice, artificial flavors, artificial sweeteners, and anything labeled partially hydrogenated (another word for trans fat).

Starch Guard

A product can claim "trans fat-free" if a single serving contains less than 0.49 grams of trans fat. Any "partially hydrogenated" ingredient is a trans fat, no matter what the nutrition facts box states.

Another significant ingredient to avoid is high-fructose corn syrup (HFCS). Unlike other sweeteners, HFCS does not stimulate the pancreas to produce insulin while traveling intact to the liver to be stored as fat. Without the secretion of insulin, the brain never receives the signal to turn off the hunger switch. By ingesting HFCS, fat storage is increased without satisfying the appetite. Many popular brand-name beverages, breads, baked goods, and ice creams contain this dangerous ingredient.

Nitrates, preservatives used to increase shelf life in processed meats (packaged deli meats and canned meats), have been linked to cancer. Sodium or potassium benzoate is often used as a preservative in soft drinks, iced teas, and other packaged foods. When combined with vitamin C (ascorbic acid), which is used in many of the same products, benzene—a chemical linked to leukemia—can form.

The crux of understanding ingredients is that simpler is usually better. If you don't recognize the ingredient, it probably isn't good for you. Examples include evaporated cane juice, which is another term for refined sugar, and FD&C Blue No. 1, which is an artificial coloring. This rule also holds true for ingredients that you are unable to pronounce. Examples include acesulfame potassium, an artificial sweetener, and monosodium glutamate, a flavor enhancer that may cause neurological damage. You also have to beware of names of other flours that are just wheat flour in disguise. Examples include bread flour, cake flour, pastry flour, all-purpose flour, and high-gluten flour.

What If I Have Gluten Intolerance (Celiac Disease)?

Celiac Disease or gluten intolerance is a disorder of the digestive system that damages the small intestine. This damage occurs because of an abnormal reaction to gluten, a protein found in wheat as well as several other grains, such as rye and barley. The reaction or inflammatory response occurs upon ingestion of gluten and interferes with the absorption of certain nutrients, vitamins, and minerals from food. It is estimated that in the United States 1 out of every 133 individuals have Celiac Disease.

To make food preparation easier for those with Celiac Disease, the recipes in this cookbook have been labeled when gluten-free. A number of food products available for retail sale are also labeled as gluten-free.

Anyone requiring a gluten-free diet needs to be extra vigilant about reading ingredients lists. Following are lists of common ingredients that contain gluten, ingredients requiring caution, and other prepared ingredients that can be "hidden" sources of gluten.

Ingredients Containing Gluten

- Barley malt
- Beer
- Bleached flour
- Brewer's yeast
- Bran
- Bread flour
- Bulgur wheat
- Cookie crumbs and dough
- Couscous
- Durum wheat
- Enriched flour
- Farina
- Germ
- Hydrolyzed wheat gluten, protein, or starch
- Kamut
- Malt extract, syrup, or flavoring
- Matzo
- Pasta

- Rye
- Seitan
- Semolina
- Spelt
- Sprouted wheat or barley
- Tabbouleh
- Teriyaki sauce
- Unbleached flour
- Whole-meal flour

Ingredients Maybe Containing Gluten (Be cautious!)

- Artificial and natural colors
- Artificial and natural flavors
- Baking powder
- Dextrins
- Emulsifiers
- Enzymes
- Food starch
- Glucose syrup
- Hydrolyzed plant or vegetable protein
- Hydrogenated starch
- Maltose
- Modified food starch
- Non-dairy creamer
- Protein hydrolysates
- Seasonings
- Soba noodles

- Soy sauce

- Vegetable broth, gum, protein, or starch

Hidden Gluten Sources

- Baked beans (in tomato sauce)

- Blue cheese (contains bread crumbs)

- Imitation crab meat (wheat based)

- Mustard (can contain gluten)

- Processed and luncheon meats (contain fillers)

- Salad dressings (added flour)

- Sausage (contains wheat)

- Sauces (often thickened with flour)

- Spices (added flour)

Just the Facts: The Nutrition Facts Box

The nutrition facts box is the road map for selecting the best foods. All packaged foods come with this information. Learn to navigate through the nutritional facts, and you're on your way to good food choices.

The nutrition facts label is divided into three parts: serving information, nutritional information, and vitamin and mineral content.

For starters, you'll find the serving size and the servings per container indicated. This indicates just how many portions each food package contains. For most, confusion arises when foods sold individually contain more than a single serving. Soft drinks, energy drinks, and sodas in small bottles are often two or more servings per container. The nutritional information on the label only reflects one serving. Many products that appear to be individual sized may actually contain two or more servings, leading you to consume many more calories and grams of sugar than you may have originally believed.

Nutrition Facts

Serving Size 1 cup (228g)
Servings Per Container 2

Amount Per Serving

Calories 250	Calories from Fat 110

	% Daily Value*
Total Fat 12g	18%
Saturated Fat 3g	15%
Trans Fat 1.5g	
Cholesterol 30mg	10%
Sodium 470mg	20%
Total Carbohydrate 31g	10%
Dietary Fiber 0g	0%
Sugars 5g	
Protein 5g	

Vitamin A	4%
Vitamin C	2%
Calcium	20%
Iron	4%

* Percent Daily Values are based on a 2,000 calorie diet. Your Daily Values may be higher or lower depending on your calorie needs:

	Calories:	2,000	2,500
Total Fat	Less than	65g	80g
Sat Fat	Less than	20g	25g
Cholesterol	Less than	300mg	300mg
Sodium	Less than	2,400mg	2,400mg
Total Carbohydrate		300g	375g
Dietary Fiber		25g	30g

Next, the nutritional information gives the amount of nutrients contained within a packaged food. On the left side of the label is the amount of each nutrient in grams, and on the right side is the percentage of daily recommended requirements based on a 2,000-calorie diet. On the bottom of the label is listed the recommended amount of total fat, saturated fat, cholesterol, sodium, total carbohydrate, and dietary fiber an individual needs each day—all based on a 2,000-calorie diet.

The nutritional information shares the calorie count, or the amount of energy provided in one serving of the food or drink. Following is information about the fat, carbohydrate, protein, sodium, and cholesterol content. Fat and carbohydrates are divided into subgroups. Total fat is subcategorized by saturated fat and trans fat. (Remember that all trans fats are unhealthy, and the foods you purchase should be devoid of trans fat.) Total carbohydrate is also subdivided by dietary fiber and sugar. Choose foods that contain more dietary fiber and less sugar.

XXXX **No-Flour Power** _____

Saturated fat and trans fat are typically the only fats accounted for on the food label, and only if the product contains more than 0.5 grams of these fats per serving. Because of this, it is important to read the ingredient list to receive "full disclosure." Examples of saturated fats include butter, coconut oil, and palm oil. Trans fats are often identified by the phrase "partially hydrogenated." Monounsaturated and polyunsaturated fats do not appear on the labels but equal the difference between total fat and trans and saturated fat.

Likewise, dietary fiber and sugar are the only carbohydrates accounted for on a food label and only if the product contains more than 0.5 grams of these carbohydrates per serving. Examples of sugars include molasses, high-fructose corn syrup, and dextrose. Examples of dietary fibers include wheat bran, cellulose, and xanthan gum. The difference between the total carbohydrate and sugar and dietary fiber represents all other carbohydrates.

Finally, the label lists four essential vitamins and minerals: vitamin A, vitamin C, calcium, and iron. The percentage to the right of these nutrients is the amount of your daily requirement the food contains per serving based on a 2,000-calorie diet. Some foods provide information for additional nutrients, vitamins, and minerals, especially when it's to their advantage.

Nutritional Analysis Application

As you read through the recipes in this book, you'll see each is accompanied by a nutritional profile. The nutrition analysis is provided to help you decide how each recipe best fits your daily dietary requirements. Emphasis is placed on creating a dish rich in protein and fiber with minimal sodium content. All are great options within a healthy, well-balanced diet. You'll find no trans fats, no added refined sugar, and no evaporated cane juice. Great alternatives to flour are called for, allowing you to enjoy the foods you love while benefitting from a more healthful lifestyle. Following is an example of one of the nutrition profiles in the book.

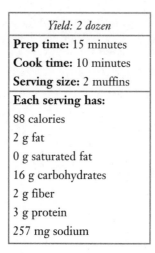

Yield: 2 dozen

Prep time: 15 minutes

Cook time: 10 minutes

Serving size: 2 muffins

Each serving has:

88 calories

2 g fat

0 g saturated fat

16 g carbohydrates

2 g fiber

3 g protein

257 mg sodium

As with the nutrition facts box, the nutrition analysis alongside each recipe in this cookbook supplies the serving size and the number of servings for the recipe. The information provided should be used as a guideline. Slight differences in exact ingredients and preparation methods may result in altered nutrient amounts. A food's nutrient values can vary by season, grower, and location. For example, recipes calling for fresh tomatoes in this book have been computed by using the year-round average for the ingredient. Summer-grown tomatoes may be more nutrient-rich.

When a recipe offers an alternative ingredient or variation, these aren't considered in the nutrition summary. The first listed ingredient is used in the calculation. As you may or may not choose to follow any suggested serving accompaniments offered at the end of some recipes, these proposals aren't taken into account either. In the same fashion, when a recipe offers a range of servings and/or a range for an ingredient amount, the nutrition analysis is figured on the first serving size and/or the first ingredient amount.

Some recipes included in this cookbook may be nutritionally sound for every day, whereas others should be considered once-in-a-while foods. These other foods include several of the desserts that may have a higher sugar count and some of the pasta dishes that have a higher carbohydrate count. Use the nutrition analysis to make the best choices for your needs.

The Least You Need to Know

- Whenever partially hydrogenated oil appears in an ingredients list, the food contains harmful trans fat.

- Foods are likely more nutritionally sound if you easily recognize their ingredients.

- All important information provided by a nutrition facts box is based on a single serving.

- Nutritional summaries are guidelines to help you decide which foods best fit your dietary needs.

5

Getting the Grist of It

In This Chapter

- ◆ Ingredient choices you can tailor to your dietary requirements
- ◆ Flour alternatives with nutrients your body needs
- ◆ Vitamins and minerals found in flour substitutions

After you decide to remove wheat-based flours from your diet to capture the health benefits, you don't want to leave a gaping hole in your eating habits. Fortunately, eliminating flour doesn't mean deprivation.

More nutrients and a greater depth of flavor can be found when you know what flour alternatives are available. Shopping the health-food section of the supermarket rather than the baking aisle will transform your kitchen, as well as how good you look and feel.

Sifting Out Better Flours

Now is the opportunity to utilize your newfound nutritional knowledge and choose alternatives to flour that help stabilize blood glucose and prevent waistline expansion. The first step is selecting food products that are nutritionally well-balanced, containing adequate amounts of the right fiber, protein, and fat.

Fiber Content

Remember that dietary fiber isn't digested in the intestines and doesn't have a caloric impact on the body. This fiber is able to slow the absorption of sugar, creating more stable blood glucose levels. Fiber provides satiety for fewer calories.

The best alternatives to flour with the highest fiber levels are as follows:

Words to Digest

Ground coconut is a low-carbohydrate flour substitute that contains the mineral manganese.

- *Ground coconut*
- Flaxseed meal
- Ground fava beans
- Ground chia seeds
- Ground garbanzo beans

Protein Content

Without protein, the body is unable to maintain proper cell and tissue function. This vital raw material comes from the amino acids that bind together to form proteins. Nine of these amino acids are called essential, not being produced by the body; they must be provided in the daily diet. Two of our flour alternatives—quinoa and amaranth—are two of the best vegetable sources of these important building blocks.

Overall, the best alternatives to flour with the highest protein levels are the following:

- Ground fava beans
- Almond meal
- Ground garbanzo beans
- Flaxseed meal
- Steel-cut oats

Fat Content

Fat is critical for keeping the body functioning efficiently. When choosing fats, they should be natural and not include the dangerous trans fats. Instead, fats should be comprised of significant levels of monounsaturated fats and omega-3 fatty acids. Two excellent choices are ground chia seeds and flaxseed meal. They are considered *super-foods* because of their elevated levels of omega-3 fatty acids, which carry with them heart-healthy and anti-inflammatory properties.

> **Words to Digest** _____
>
> A **superfood** is a food that provides health benefits above and beyond basic macronutrients. These foods may help lower our risk of developing disease such as heart disease, type 2 diabetes, and cancer.

The recommended flour substitutes with the highest levels of good fats are the following:

- Ground hazelnuts
- Almond meal
- Flaxseed meal
- Ground chia seeds
- Ground coconut

Flour Alternatives

Wheat-based flours are staples in modern cooking and baking. Eating flour-free requires replacing commonplace flours and flour products with suitable alternatives. Other ground grains, ground nuts, and ground beans can be substituted for a more healthful diet.

Almond Meal

Ground almond meal is a byproduct of whole or blanched almonds with a consistency similar to cornmeal. This ingredient is traditionally used in almond macaroons, as a cake or pie filling, and as the primary ingredient in marzipan. Almond meal has become a popular ingredient in baking low-sugar or low-carbohydrate products. Calorie-dense, it adds both moistness and a rich, nutty taste to foods.

Because almond meal tastes generally neutral, it's an excellent substitute for wheat-based flours. Almond meal can also be used to thicken sauces, as a base for pie crusts, and as a key ingredient in cookie batter.

Nutritionally, almond meal is a superfood providing many essential vitamins and minerals. Additionally, it's a good source of fiber and a heart-healthy monounsaturated fat.

Almond meal is an excellent source of vitamins and minerals, including the following:

- Copper
- Magnesium
- Phosphorus
- Riboflavin (vitamin B2)
- Vitamin E

Flaxseed Meal

Ground flaxseed meal is comprised of whole and ground flaxseeds available in either a golden or brown color. The color variation is due to different versions of the same seed with identical nutritional benefits. Golden flaxseeds are grown primarily in North Dakota and Montana while brown flaxseeds are grown in the prairie provinces of Canada.

Because most flaxseeds' carbohydrates are fiber-based, the ground meal is a great alternative for people looking to limit their intake of sugars and starches. Its robust, nutty flavor makes it a good choice for baked goods.

Flaxseeds are another superfood containing an abundance of healthy fats, minerals, and vitamins. Flaxseeds are rich in alpha linolenic acid (ALA), an omega-3 fatty acid that converts to eicosapentaenoic acid (EPA). EPA is found in fish oils. Flaxseed meal is an excellent alternative for individuals who cannot include fish or fish oil in their diets.

An excellent source of insoluble and soluble fibers, flaxseed meal is the best plant source of lignan phytonutrients. This type of fiber source is a powerful antioxidant that helps prevent premature aging and disease, lower cholesterol, regulate the bowels, and stabilize blood glucose levels.

With flaxseed meal's combination of healthy fats and dietary fiber, adding it to recipes produces greater satiety with fewer calories and better blood glucose control.

A nutritional powerhouse, flaxseed meal contains the following vitamins and minerals:

- Copper
- Folate
- Magnesium
- Manganese
- Phosphorus
- Thiamine (vitamin B1)
- Vitamin B6

Ground Coconut

Ground coconut is produced from dried coconut meat. A combination of coconut oil, dietary fiber, water, protein, and carbohydrates, ground coconut is ideal for baking because of its rich texture and natural sweetness. Use it in breads, cakes, pies, desserts, cookies, pancakes, and waffles.

Fifty-eight percent dietary fiber, ground coconut helps promote satiety and keep blood glucose levels stable. It has the highest fiber content of any flour alternative.

Ground Fava Beans

Native to North Africa and Southwest Asia, the fava bean is also called the broad bean. Large and brown, favas are often considered one of the better-tasting members of the bean family because of its mild taste. Traditionally, this bean is used in Mediterranean and Chinese dishes. This mild taste, in contrast to many other beans, makes it a superb substitute for white flour.

Ground fava beans are an excellent source of L-dopa, an amino acid that is converted to dopamine and helpful in treating Parkinson's disease. Research also indicates that fava beans may protect against malaria.

The super fava bean contains vitamins and minerals that include the following:

♦ Copper

♦ Folate

♦ Iron

♦ Magnesium

♦ Manganese

♦ Phosphorus

♦ Thiamine (vitamin B1)

Chia Seeds

Ground chia seeds are an ancient Mexican food dating back more than 4,600 years. The seed is ground into *pinole*, a meal used in baked goods and porridge. Ground chia seeds are very similar to flaxseed. They're a good nonfish source of omega-3 fatty acids and soluble fiber. With exceptional amounts of antioxidants, chia seeds enjoy healthy properties that help slow the absorption of glucose, benefit the heart, and prevent premature aging and disease. Best of all, chia seeds can help you become satiated on fewer calories because of their ability to absorb up to 10 times their weight in water.

The dynamic chia seed contains the following minerals:

♦ Boron

♦ Calcium

♦ Manganese

♦ Phosphorus

Ground Hazelnuts

Hazelnuts, another ancient food, have been consumed for more than 5,000 years. Also known as filberts, hazelnuts are considered a super nut just like almonds, pecans, and walnuts. Hazelnuts are differentiated by their rich flavor and upscale appeal. Their indulgent nature and wonderful sweet flavor make them a great choice for all baked goods, especially muffins, cakes, and cookies.

This nutritional powerhouse is high in heart-healthy monounsaturated fats while providing plenty of fiber and protein. A strong antioxidant, the hazelnut contains one of the highest amounts of proanthocyandins, a phytochemical that decreases the risk of cancer and heart disease. In addition, these compounds may lessen the incidence of urinary tract infections and blood clotting.

Hazelnuts contain the following vitamins and minerals:

◆ Copper

◆ Folate

◆ Iron

◆ Magnesium

◆ Manganese

◆ Thiamine (vitamin B1)

◆ Vitamin B6

◆ Vitamin E

Konjac Noodles

Konjac noodles, also known as Shirataki noodles, are made from konjac glucomannan. Glucomannan is a soluble dietary fiber derived from the konjac plant. These noodles are used in traditional Chinese and Japanese foods.

With their high fiber content, konjac noodles slow down the digestion of glucose and create satiety without additional calories. These noodles contain no fat, sugar, starch, or protein. Because the fiber is soluble, the noodles are devoid of any vitamins and minerals.

Ground Garbanzo Beans

Garbanzo beans, also known as chickpeas or ceci beans (among other names), originated in the Middle East more than 7,000 years ago. This versatile legume is a common ingredient in Middle Eastern and Indian favorites, such as hummus, falafel, and curry. Usually beige in color, garbanzo beans can also be black, green, red, or brown. With their nutlike taste and buttery texture, ground garbanzo beans can substitute for flour in baked goods and breads.

Because garbanzo beans are rich in protein and fiber, they're helpful in improving digestion, delaying the absorption of sugar, stabilizing blood glucose levels, and lowering cholesterol.

Garbanzo beans contain the following vitamins and minerals:

- Copper
- Folate
- Iron
- Magnesium
- Manganese
- Pantothenic acid
- Potassium
- Thiamine (vitamin B1)
- Vitamin B6
- Zinc

> **XXXX** **No-Flour Power** _____
>
> Several recipes in this cookbook call for ground garbanzo beans and ground fava beans in a single measurement. Look for the combined ground beans product where you purchase other flour substitutes. Alternatively, mix your own blend, beginning with a half-and-half mixture and adjusting it to your personal preference.

Amaranth

Amaranth is an ancient grain dating back to the Aztecs, who considered it sacred. Amaranth is a plant that is both a high-protein grain and a leafy vegetable. As a grain, it's a popular substitute for flour in gluten-free recipes. Use it in breads, noodles, pancakes, cereals, and cookies.

Amaranth is a good source of protein and dietary fiber. Because of its high content of essential amino acids required for cell and brain function, amaranth is a great source of vegetable protein.

Amaranth, an Aztec superfood, contains the following vitamins and minerals:

◆ Calcium

◆ Folate

◆ Iron

◆ Magnesium

◆ Manganese

◆ Phosphorus

◆ Selenium

◆ Vitamin B6

◆ Zinc

Sorghum

Sorghum, first used in Africa 3,000 years ago, is a popular cereal grain because of its capability to grow in semi-arid climates with limited water supply. The grain is either red or pale yellow in color. Cooked as porridge, sorghum is a common breakfast food. It's also a typical flour substitute in gluten-free cooking. Sorghum must be blended with other flour substitutes, however, to prevent baked goods from being dry and gritty.

Sorghum provides some protein and fiber, which help balance its carbohydrate content. Its major health benefit is from large amounts of policonosal, a strong anti-oxidant that may lower cholesterol and improve heart health.

The special sorghum grain contains the following:

◆ Iron

◆ Phosphorus

◆ Thiamine (vitamin B1)

Quinoa

Quinoa isn't a grain but actually a relative of dark green, leafy vegetables. An ancient food once known as the "gold of the Incas," the cooked product gives off a nutty flavor with a nice, crunchy texture. Quinoa works as a great grain substitute in almost any dish.

Quinoa is one of the few foods that provide a complete protein profile, containing all nine essential amino acids. It's also a great source of antioxidants with two types of phytonutrients: plant lignans and phenolics, which are thought to protect against some hormonal cancers (i.e., breast cancer) and heart disease.

Quinoa contains the following vitamins and minerals:

- Copper
- Folate
- Iron
- Magnesium
- Manganese
- Phosphorus
- Riboflavin (vitamin B2)
- Thiamine (vitamin B1)
- Vitamin B6
- Zinc

Steel-Cut Oats

Steel-cut oats, also called Irish or Scottish oats, are natural, unrefined oat *groats* processed with a minimal amount of heat, and not rolled. Because of their manufacturing process, they require more time to cook than rolled oats and provide a chewy texture. These oats are golden in color and are mostly used in cereal-based products.

Words to Digest

Groat is the term for a cereal grain such as oats, wheat, or buckwheat that only has the outer shell or coating removed.

Steel-cut oats are a good source of soluble fiber and protein. They also contain a significant level of a special fiber, beta-glucan. Research has shown beta-glucan to affect the immune system by increasing the body's ability to ward off bacterial infections. Beta-glucan also lowers cholesterol levels and minimizes blood glucose spikes in diabetics.

Beneficial steel-cut oats contain the following:

◆ Copper

◆ Iron

◆ Magnesium

◆ Manganese

◆ Phosphorus

◆ Thiamine (vitamin B1)

◆ Zinc

Stone-Ground Cornmeal

Stone-ground cornmeal is a byproduct of dried corn kernels. Cornmeal is either stone-ground or steel-ground, depending on how it is milled. The advantage of stone-ground cornmeal is that it retains more of the corn's hull and germ, the source of fiber and nutrients. Cornmeal comes in several colors—yellow, white, or blue—according to the variety of the corn used. Cornmeal is often served as a hot breakfast cereal or used in baking breads, pancakes, and muffins.

Cornmeal has high levels of fiber, which aids in satiety, blood glucose stability, and healthy digestion. It's rich in carotenoids, an antioxidant that may lower the risk of developing cancer.

Stone-ground cornmeal contains the following:

◆ Magnesium

◆ Manganese

◆ Thiamine (vitamin B1)

◆ Vitamin E

Brown Rice Meal

Brown rice is produced by removing the outermost layer of the rice kernel, the hull, which contains most of its nutritional value. When rice kernels are completely milled to white rice, almost all nutrients are lost, including all the dietary fiber and essential fatty acids. Rice is a very popular food representing as much as 50 percent of daily calories in many countries around the world. Brown rice meal is used as a flour substitute to make breads, cookies, and muffins.

Because of its fiber content, brown rice meal has been shown to decrease the risk of heart disease while helping to manage weight and prevent diabetes. It contains plant lignans, which studies have shown protects the body against cancer and heart disease.

This whole grain contains the following vitamins and minerals:

◆ Magnesium

◆ Manganese

◆ Niacin

◆ Phosphorus

◆ Vitamin B6

The Least You Need to Know

◆ Healthy fats, fibers, and proteins can enhance your foods when you substitute for flour.

◆ A variety of ground whole grains, beans, and nuts can supply the texture you need when replacing flour.

◆ Flour-based, starchy products—such as pastas, breads, instant oats, and more—can be swapped out for prepared or purchased foods made from more healthful ingredients.

◆ Eliminating flour from your diet can even out blood glucose levels and thwart waistline expansion.

Part 2

Better Breakfasts, Brunches, and Breads

Breakfast—we all know it's the most important meal of the day. So why is traditional early-morning fare full of flour and unhealthful sugars?

You can start your day off right by making good decisions at the breakfast table. Preparing flour-free morning meals provides the best nutrients and high energy you need to get through your day. A few subtle changes to typical ingredients will put you on the path to a more healthful, productive day.

Chapter 6

Good-Start Breakfasts and Brunches

In This Chapter

- ◆ Great grains to rev up your metabolism

- ◆ Fabulous fruits to sweeten your morning

- ◆ Everyone's favorite eggs

Jump-start your day with a well-balanced breakfast. Remember, the first meal in the morning sets the pace for the rest of the day. By focusing on nutrient-dense foods rather than opting for morning meals packed with flour and sugar, you avoid the blood sugar roller coaster. You'll improve your metabolism and keep your internal engine running smoothly.

Making a Difference at Daybreak

The breakfast recipes in this chapter provide a new perspective on traditionally flour-full, sugar-stuffed morning selections. Oatmeal, pancakes, yogurt, and toast can still be savored—just without flour or added sugar. Steel-cut oats, stone-ground cornmeal, sprouted-grain bread, Greek yogurt, *agave nectar*—the healthful ingredients list goes on and on. You can't help but think of delicious new ways to incorporate these foods into your morning routine.

Words to Digest

Agave nectar, or agave syrup, is a natural sweetener derived from the agave plant grown in Mexico. The syrup's uses include sweetening beverages, supplying sweetness in cooking, and substituting for sugary breakfast toppings. Look for raw agave nectar, a minimally processed syrup not heated higher than 118°F to protect the natural enzymes.

Choosing a more healthful start to your day is simple. Stock up your pantry with nutritious ingredients and wield your creativity in the kitchen!

Apple and Cinnamon Steel-Cut Oatmeal

The sweet fragrance of apple and cinnamon tempt you to the slightly nutty taste of this chewy-textured breakfast treat.

½ cup steel-cut oats

¼ tsp. ground cinnamon

1½ cups boiling water

1 medium Gala apple, cored and chopped

¼ cup fat-free milk

1 TB. honey

Yield: 2 servings
Prep time: 2 minutes
Cook time: 27 to 33 minutes
Serving size: 1 cup
Each serving has:
277 calories
3 g fat
1 g saturated fat
55 g carbohydrates
7 g fiber
7 g protein
21 mg sodium

1. Add steel-cut oats to a small nonstick saucepan and place over medium heat; cook for 2 to 3 minutes, stirring frequently, or until toasted and fragrant. Stir in cinnamon.

2. Carefully pour in boiling water. Stir in chopped apple. Cover, reduce heat to low, and simmer for 20 minutes, stirring occasionally, or until most of the liquid is absorbed.

3. Remove from heat. Stir in milk and honey. Let stand, uncovered, for 5 to 10 minutes or until desired consistency is reached.

Variation: Any cooking apple you have in your fruit bowl can be used in this recipe.

XXXX No-Flour Power

Cooking apples resist turning to mush when heated. In addition to Galas, some good choices to try are the Cortland, Granny Smith, Jonathan, Northern Spy, Pippin, Rome Beauty, and Winesap.

Overnight Milk-and-Honey Steel-Cut Oatmeal

The perfect balance of creamy and chewy can be indulged in without the time-consuming morning preparation.

Yield: 1 serving
Prep time: 10 minutes
Chill time: 8 hours
Cook time: 12 minutes
Serving size: 1 cup
Each serving has:
277 calories
3 g fat
1 g saturated fat
48 g carbohydrates
4 g fiber
14 g protein
126 mg sodium

¼ **cup steel-cut oats**   ½ **TB. honey**

1 cup fat-free milk

1. Combine steel-cut oats and milk in a small nonstick saucepan. Heat over high heat, stirring often, for about 5 minutes or until milk bubbles actively at the edge of the saucepan. Stir constantly when milk is hot, scraping the bottom of the saucepan to prevent milk from scorching and boiling over.

2. Reduce heat to low. Simmer for 2 minutes, stirring slowly to scrape the bottom of the saucepan to prevent milk from scorching.

3. Remove from heat. Stir often to prevent milk from sticking to the bottom of the saucepan and to cool, about 8 minutes. Cover and refrigerate overnight.

4. Uncover and heat over high heat for about 5 minutes or until milk actively bubbles at the edge of the saucepan, stirring often and scraping the bottom of the saucepan to prevent milk from scorching.

5. Turn off heat, stir in honey, and serve hot.

Variation: Serve this oatmeal as prepared or add your favorite oatmeal toppings, such as fresh blueberries, sliced bananas, raisins, or ground flaxseed meal.

For Good Measure

Although old-fashioned rolled oats and steel-cut oats are nutritionally comparable, steel-cut oats are minimally processed. Rolled oats are manufactured by steaming and rolling the whole oat groats. Steel-cut oats are whole oat groats that have been cut into two or three pieces by steel blades, allowing for their chewy (never mushy) texture.

Sautéed Apples Atop Cinnamon-Raisin Sprouted-Grain Bread

Start your day with a delicious but more healthful choice for cheddar-topped apple pie.

1 tsp. unsalted butter

½ medium Granny Smith apple, cored and thinly sliced

¼ cup 100 percent natural fresh-pressed apple juice

1 slice cinnamon-raisin sprouted-grain bread, toasted

1 thin slice white cheddar cheese

Yield: 1 serving
Prep time: 1 minute
Cook time: 8 minutes
Serving size: 1 slice
Each serving has:
308 calories
12 g fat
7 g saturated fat
43 g carbohydrates
5 g fiber
8 g protein
191 mg sodium

1. In a 9-inch nonstick skillet over medium heat, melt butter. Add apple slices, and stir to coat. Cook, stirring often, for 2 minutes or until apples soften and butter bubbles. Carefully pour in apple juice, and stir to coat apples. Cook, stirring occasionally, for 5 minutes or until apples are tender and the skillet is nearly dry.

2. Turn out apples onto toasted cinnamon-raisin bread. Top with cheese slice, pressing onto apples to melt. Serve immediately.

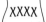

No-Flour Power _____

Flourless sprouted-grain breads can most often be found in your grocer's freezer section. If your supermarket maintains a natural foods department, check the freezer case there.

Kickin' Scrambled Eggs with Horseradish and Chives

Heat things up at the breakfast table with the addition of biting homemade horseradish in velvety eggs. This recipe is gluten-free.

Yield: 1 serving
Prep time: 1 minute
Cook time: 4 minutes
Serving size: 2 eggs
Each serving has:
153 calories
10 g fat
3 g saturated fat
3 g carbohydrates
0 g fiber
13 g protein
407 mg sodium

2 large eggs

2 TB. cold water

2 tsp. Simple Two-Ingredient Horseradish (recipe later in this chapter), or more to taste

2 tsp. chopped fresh chives

Pinch fine sea salt

Pinch freshly ground black pepper

1. Heat a small nonstick skillet over medium to medium-low heat for 1 minute. When the skillet is hot, coat with cooking spray.

2. Meanwhile, in a small bowl, whisk eggs until lemon-colored. Whisk in cold water. Pour egg mixture into the hot skillet. Cook for 2 minutes without stirring, or until underside of eggs is set.

3. Add Simple Two-Ingredient Horseradish, chives, sea salt, and black pepper. Stir set eggs up from the bottom, allowing un-cooked eggs to run into the skillet. Cook and stir for 2 minutes or until eggs are set (160°F on a food thermometer).

4. Remove from heat and serve immediately.

 For Good Measure

Sea salt is available in coarse and fine grains which, because unrefined, may contain other minerals such as magnesium, iron, and calcium. Table salt is sodium chloride with additives that may include sugar.

Simple Two-Ingredient Horseradish

Savor the piquant flavor of fresh horseradish that saves on the sugars, starches, and salts often found in commercially prepared horseradishes. This recipe is gluten-free.

1 (10- to 11-inch) horseradish root	**½ cup white vinegar, or as needed**

Yield: 1 cup
Prep time: 10 minutes
Serving size: 2 teaspoons
Each serving has:
6 calories
0 g fat
0 g saturated fat
1 g carbohydrates
0 g fiber
0 g protein
0 mg sodium

1. Peel brown skin from horseradish root with a vegetable peeler, and chop horseradish root coarsely with a sharp knife. (You should have about 1 cup chopped horseradish root.)

2. Place horseradish root in a blender. Cover and blend on high for 5 seconds or until roughly shredded. Carefully tip up the lid's cap to pour in vinegar a little at a time while grating on high speed. Blend for 3 minutes or until mixture is creamy. Stop the blender to scrape down sides as needed.

3. Spoon horseradish into a small glass jar. Close lid tightly and refrigerate. Use within 3 to 4 months.

Starch Guard

We recommend preparing homemade horseradish in a well-ventilated area. Also, take care not to hold your face over or breathe directly over the open blender. Fresh horseradish can bring tears to your eyes and take your breath away.

Strawberries, Flax, and Toasted Pecans Parfait

Protein-packed, thick-textured Greek yogurt is the perfect vehicle for the sweetened berries making a creamy, fruity start to your day with an added nutty crunch. This recipe is gluten-free.

Yield: 1 serving
Prep time: 5 minutes
Chill time: 8 hours
Cook time: 3 minutes
Serving size: 1½ cups
Each serving has:
330 calories
13 g fat
1 g saturated fat
38 g carbohydrates
7 g fiber
16 g protein
48 mg sodium

1 cup sliced fresh strawberries

1 TB. honey

½ cup fat-free plain Greek yogurt

1 TB. ground flaxseed meal

2 TB. chopped pecans

1. Combine ¼ cup strawberries and honey in a small bowl. With the back of a fork, mash strawberries until mixture is syrupy. Stir in yogurt until blended.

2. In a 12-ounce parfait dish or glass, layer ⅓ of yogurt mixture, 1 teaspoon ground flaxseed meal, and ½ of remaining strawberries. Repeat layering. Spoon in remaining yogurt mixture and sprinkle remaining 1 teaspoon ground flaxseed meal on top. Cover and chill overnight.

3. In a small, dry skillet, toast chopped pecans for 3 minutes, stirring frequently, or until lightly browned and fragrant. Remove from heat. Store in an airtight container or prepare just before serving. Sprinkle on top of parfait.

Starch Guard

Watch the pecans closely as they toast, remembering to stir them frequently. Nuts are quick to burn.

Fruity Flax Breakfast Smoothie

This fast-fix start for your morning sips thick and creamy, cool and fresh. This recipe is gluten-free.

1 cup cubed cantaloupe

¾ cup halved fresh strawberries

½ cup fat-free plain Greek yogurt

¼ cup 100 percent natural fresh-pressed apple juice

2 TB. ground flaxseed meal

½ TB. honey

½ tsp. vanilla extract

12 small ice cubes

Yield: 1 serving		
Prep time: 2 minutes		
Serving size: 2¼ cups		
Each serving has:		
310 calories		
5 g fat		
0 g saturated fat		
48 g carbohydrates		
8 g fiber		
17 g protein		
64 mg sodium		

1. Add cantaloupe, strawberries, yogurt, apple juice, ground flaxseed meal, honey, and vanilla extract to a blender. Cover and blend on high for 30 seconds or until blended.

2. Open the cap on the blender's lid and add ice cubes 1 at a time until crushed (about 30 seconds). Stop the blender. Pour into a tall glass or a commuter cup for an on-the-go breakfast.

Variation: You can substitute your favorite fresh fruits. Try peaches, pineapple, raspberries, and more in the same proportions.

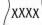

No-Flour Power

If your favorite fruits aren't in season and you need to substitute with their frozen counterparts, be sure to choose the unsweetened packages.

Rustic Johnnycakes

Wake up your taste buds with these crisp-skinned, hearty corn-flavored pancakes. This recipe is gluten-free.

Yield: 3 servings
Prep time: 5 minutes
Cook time: 4 minutes per batch
Serving size: 2 johnny-cakes
Each serving has:
235 calories
9 g fat
5 g saturated fat
33 g carbohydrates
3 g fiber
5 g protein
409 mg sodium

1 cup stone-ground yellow cornmeal

½ tsp. fine sea salt

2 TB. unsalted butter, cut into small pieces

½ cup fat-free milk

2 TB. boiling water or as needed

1. In a medium bowl, stir together yellow cornmeal and sea salt. Using a pastry blender or 2 butter knives, cut butter into cornmeal mixture until crumbly.

2. Pour in milk, and stir until dry ingredients are moistened. Add boiling water, 1 tablespoon at a time, to thin batter.

3. Meanwhile, heat a large nonstick skillet over medium heat. When hot, coat with cooking spray.

4. Spoon batter into the hot skillet by heaping spoonfuls, and, using the back of the spoon, flatten batter into about 4-inch circles. Cook johnnycakes for 2 minutes or until edges are cooked and crisp. Using a spatula, flip johnnycakes and cook for 2 minutes more or until golden brown on undersides. Repeat with remaining batter. Top with agave nectar, warmed fruit spread, or a pat of butter, if desired.

For Good Measure

Stone-ground cornmeal utilizes the whole grain so that the corn germ's oils and vitamins are ground into the corn-meal.

Basic Crepes Batter

Even more delicate than traditional crepes, these thin pancakes offer a hint of nutty flavor. This recipe is gluten-free.

½ **cup ground almond meal**

½ **cup stone-ground brown rice**

¼ **tsp. fine sea salt**

1¼ **cups fat-free milk**

2 **TB. extra-virgin olive oil**

2 **large eggs**

Yield: 4 (8-inch) crepes
Prep time: 10 minutes
Chill time: 1 hour
Cook time: 12 minutes
Serving size: 1 crepe
Each serving has:
280 calories
17 g fat
2 g saturated fat
23 g carbohydrates
3 g fiber
10 g protein
212 mg sodium

1. In a medium bowl, stir together ground almond meal, stone-ground brown rice, and sea salt. While whisking, slowly pour in milk. Whisk in extra-virgin olive oil. Whisk in eggs, 1 at a time. Chill for at least 1 hour.

2. Whisk batter until well blended. Heat an 8-inch crepe pan or a nonstick skillet with an 8-inch surface over medium heat. When hot, coat with cooking spray. Whisk batter to blend again and measure ½ cup.

3. Gradually pour measured batter into the prepared crepe pan to distribute evenly. Cook for 2 minutes or until edges are cooked and top is dry.

4. Very carefully slide crepe onto a wide spatula, and gently flip back into the pan onto the other side. Cook for 1 minute or until golden brown on the underside.

5. Turn the crepe pan upside-down over a flat surface or a plate to release crepe. Let stand until cooled.

6. Keep the crepe pan off the heat. Whisk batter to blend. Return the crepe pan to the heat, and coat with cooking spray. Whisk batter to blend, and measure ½ cup.

7. Gradually pour measured batter into the prepared crepe pan to evenly distribute. Finish cooking as directed. Repeat with remaining batter. (Cooked crepes can be layered on top of each other to cool, if needed.)

8. If not serving immediately, cover and refrigerate; reheat briefly in the microwave to warm, if needed.

For Good Measure

Because this crepe batter recipe is unsweetened, you can use these crepes for both sweet and savory fillings.

Lemon-Kissed Blueberry Crepes

This creamy blueberry filling is brightened by the tangy lemon touch that complements these lightly almond-flavored crepes. This recipe is gluten-free.

Yield: 4 servings
Prep time: 5 minutes
Serving size: 1 crepe
Each serving has:
334 calories
17 g fat
2 g saturated fat
33 g carbohydrates
3 g fiber
13 g protein
224 mg sodium

⅔ **cup fresh blueberries**

4 tsp. agave nectar

½ **cup fat-free plain Greek yogurt**

1 tsp. freshly grated lemon *zest*

4 (8-inch) prepared Basic Crepes Batter (recipe earlier in this chapter) crepes

1. In a small bowl, combine ⅓ cup blueberries and agave nectar. With the back of a fork, mash blueberries until mixture is tinged purple and blueberries are broken up. Add Greek yogurt and lemon zest, and stir until blended.

2. Spoon yogurt mixture down the centers of prepared crepes, dividing equally. Fold the left side of each crepe over filling, and then fold in the right side to close each crepe. Garnish with remaining ⅓ cup blueberries to serve.

Words to Digest

Zest is the term referring to small slivers of peel, usually from a citrus fruit such as a lemon, lime, or orange. The colorful peels contain flavorful oils, but the underlying white pith is bitter-tasting.

Cinnamon-Flecked Cottage Pancakes with Red Raspberry Sauce

These thin, airy pancakes have a hint of cinnamon and are sweetened by a drizzle of melted red raspberry fruit spread. This recipe is gluten-free.

1 cup 1-percent low-fat small-curd cottage cheese

4 large eggs, at room temperature

¼ cup ground almond meal

1 tsp. ground cinnamon

⅛ tsp. fine sea salt

½ cup all-fruit seedless red raspberry spreadable fruit

Yield: 8 servings
Prep time: 2 minutes
Cook time: 5 minutes per batch
Serving size: 2 pancakes plus 1 tablespoon sauce
Each serving has:
118 calories
5 g fat
1 g saturated fat
12 g carbohydrates
1 g fiber
7 g protein
181 mg sodium

1. Heat a large nonstick skillet over medium to medium-low heat. When hot, coat with cooking spray.

2. Meanwhile, add cottage cheese and 2 eggs to a blender. Cover and blend on high for 30 seconds or until mixture is blended. Add remaining 2 eggs, ground almond meal, cinnamon, and sea salt. Cover and blend on high for 30 seconds or until all ingredients are blended. Stop to scrape down sides as needed.

3. Pour 2 tablespoons of batter into the hot skillet for each pancake. Cook for 2 to 2½ minutes or until top is bubbly and edges are dry.

4. Using a wide spatula, carefully flip each pancake. Cook for 2 minutes or until underside is browned. Cook in batches until all batter is used, coating the skillet with cooking spray between batches. Keep cooked pancakes warm in an oven set to low.

5. Meanwhile, place spreadable fruit in a small saucepan. Heat over medium heat, stirring frequently, for 2 minutes or until melted. Turn off heat. Keep warm, and drizzle over pancakes to serve.

Starch Guard

Some cornstarch is used to make cottage cheese. You'll want to read the ingredients lists to choose a version and brand that uses the least amount.

Sweet Sorghum Waffles

Start your morning off with a sweet and hearty waffle that's crisp on the outside and tender on the inside with a touch of rich nutty flavor. This recipe is gluten-free.

Yield: 8 servings
Prep time: 6 minutes
Cook time: 2 minutes
Serving size: 1 (4×4-inch) waffle
Each serving has:
142 calories
7 g fat
1 g saturated fat
15 g carbohydrates
2 g fiber
5 g protein
219 mg sodium

¾ **cup ground almond meal**

¼ **cup ground sorghum**

1 **tsp. baking soda**

Pinch fine sea salt

3 **large eggs, at room temperature**

¼ **cup honey**

2 **TB. fat-free plain yogurt**

1 **tsp. vanilla extract**

1. Preheat an 8×8 waffle iron.

2. In a medium bowl, combine ground almond meal, ground sorghum, baking soda, and sea salt.

3. In a 4-cup measuring cup, whisk eggs until lemon-colored. Add honey, and whisk until blended. Stir in yogurt and vanilla extract to blend. Gradually whisk in dry ingredients until mixed.

4. Set the waffle iron to the lightest waffle setting, and coat well with cooking spray. Quickly pour ¾ cup batter onto the waffle iron and close. Cook for 1 minute or until waffles are puffed and golden brown and release from the waffle iron. Remove immediately.

5. Coat the waffle iron with cooking spray and repeat with remaining batter. Serve hot with maple syrup, agave nectar, yogurt, or fresh fruit, as desired.

For Good Measure

Sorghum is a tropical grass that bears small, lustrous grains. The sweet sorghum plants are more popularly known for their sweet juices used to make syrup. The grain can be eaten as well and, when ground, substituted for flour.

Peaches-and-Cream-Stuffed French Toast

Elevate the homey taste of this breakfast favorite with a creamy, sweet filling that creates a delicious brunch entrée or a sandwich perfect for slicing into fingers for a buffet.

2 large eggs

⅔ cup fat-free milk

½ TB. honey

Pinch fine sea salt

¼ tsp. ground cinnamon

2 oz. Neufchâtel cheese or reduced-fat cream cheese

8 slices sprouted-grain bread

¼ cup all-fruit chunky peach spreadable fruit

Yield: 4 servings
Prep time: 5 minutes
Cook time: 10 minutes
Serving size: 1 piece
Each serving has:
300 calories
7 g fat
3 g saturated fat
45 g carbohydrates
6 g fiber
14 g protein
328 mg sodium

1. Preheat the oven to 450°F.

2. In a shallow dish, whisk eggs until lemon-colored. Whisk in milk. Add honey, and whisk until incorporated. Whisk in sea salt and cinnamon.

3. Spread ½ ounce Neufchâtel cheese on 4 bread slices. Spread 1 tablespoon spreadable fruit on remaining 4 bread slices, and place atop cheese-smeared slices to close sandwiches.

4. Dip both sides of stuffed sandwiches in egg mixture, coating thoroughly. Arrange on a large nonstick baking sheet coated with cooking spray. Bake for 10 minutes, turning halfway through baking time to brown evenly. Serve with pure maple syrup, agave nectar, or your favorite topping, as desired.

Starch Guard

Don't substitute fat-free cream cheese in your cooking if you're eliminating unnecessary additives. When manufacturers take out the fat, they pump up the product by adding sugars and starches.

Broccoli Cheddar Crustless Quiche

With the smooth taste of cheesy eggs studded with tender broccoli, you'll never miss the floury crust. This recipe is gluten-free.

Yield: 4 servings
Prep time: 10 minutes
Cook time: 40 minutes
Serving size: 1 wedge
Each serving has:
223 calories
16 g fat
9 g saturated fat
4 g carbohydrates
1 g fiber
16 g protein
422 mg sodium

1 cup small broccoli florets

¼ cup diced sweet onions

4 large eggs, at room temperature

¼ cup fat-free milk

¼ tsp. fine sea salt

¼ tsp. freshly ground black pepper

¼ tsp. paprika

1 cup shredded mild cheddar cheese

1. Preheat the oven to 350°F.

2. Place broccoli and sweet onions in a steamer basket over 1 inch of water. Cover and bring to a boil over high heat. Reduce heat to medium, and steam for 6 minutes or until tender. Remove vegetables and cool slightly.

3. In a medium bowl, whisk eggs until lemon-colored. Add milk, sea salt, black pepper, and paprika, and stir to blend. Add broccoli mixture and cheese, and stir to mix.

4. Pour mixture into an 8-inch pie plate coated with cooking spray, and evenly distribute broccoli and cheese. Bake for 30 minutes or until eggs are set and golden-brown and the temperature reads 160°F on a food thermometer.

5. Let stand for 5 minutes before cutting into wedges to serve.

For Good Measure

Cooking sprays are great at releasing your foods for easy serving and clean-up, but not all cooking sprays are created equal. Read the labels to choose the most natural, preservative-free versions. Or spray your oil of choice with an oil mister.

Asparagus and Mushroom Brown-Rice-Crusted Quiche

This hearty quiche's brown-rice crust offers a stable foundation while not distracting from the rich asparagus-flavored filling. This recipe is gluten-free.

1½ cups cooked long-grain brown rice, cooled

2 TB. plus ¼ cup shredded Parmesan cheese

4 large eggs

1½ cups 1-inch-cut fresh asparagus

1 TB. unsalted butter

½ cup chopped fresh mushrooms

¼ cup finely diced red onions

⅓ cup fat-free milk

2 TB. chopped fresh parsley

¼ tsp. fine sea salt

¼ tsp. freshly ground black pepper

Yield: 6 servings
Prep time: 12 minutes
Cook time: 1 hour
Serving size: 1 wedge
Each serving has:
160 calories
7 g fat
3 g saturated fat
15 g carbohydrates
2 g fiber
9 g protein
231 mg sodium

1. Preheat the oven to 350°F.

2. In a medium bowl, combine brown rice, 2 tablespoons Parmesan cheese, and 1 egg. Stir until well mixed. Spoon into an 8-inch pie plate coated with cooking spray.

3. Using the back of a fork, press the mixture on the bottom and up the side of the pie plate to cover completely. Bake for 15 minutes.

4. Meanwhile, place asparagus in a steamer basket over 1 inch of water. Cover and bring to a boil over high heat. Reduce heat to medium, and steam for 5 minutes or until tender.

5. Meanwhile, in a small skillet over medium heat, melt butter. Stir in mushrooms and red onions. Cook for 5 minutes, stirring often, or until mushrooms are browned and red onions are softened. Remove from heat. Transfer asparagus to the skillet, and stir to combine.

6. In the medium bowl, whisk 3 eggs until lemon-colored. Stir in milk. Add ¼ cup Parmesan cheese, parsley, sea salt, and black pepper, and stir to mix.

7. Remove crust from oven. Transfer asparagus mixture into crust, distributing evenly. Carefully pour in egg mixture. Bake for 45 minutes or until eggs are set and top is puffed and golden-brown.

8. Let stand for 5 minutes before serving. Cut into wedges and serve hot or at room temperature.

No-Flour Power

To prepare fresh asparagus, trim the woody stem ends. Hold the asparagus stalk at the stem end and the middle. Snap the stalk, allowing it to break at its natural breaking point (a couple inches or so from the end). Discard the woody stem ends and wash the stalks.

Anytime Muffins and Quick Breads

In This Chapter

- ◆ Tasty baked goods without a scoop of flour
- ◆ Single-serving muffins in your favorite flavors
- ◆ Crowd-pleasing quick bread loaves that everyone loves

When you think of baking a batch of yummy muffins or mixing together a quick bread batter, you probably reach for the flour canister. With your flour scoop empty, though, can you still indulge in these tasty treats? Of course!

So let your taste buds rejoice! With a few savvy substitutes, the luscious aromas of baked goods can be wafting from your oven in no time.

The Big Chill

All-purpose flour and its many relations are a boon for food manufacturers. With all the soon-to-spoil bits of the grain removed, a sack of flour enjoys a long shelf life.

The flour substitutes called for in these recipes, however, are wholesome whole grains and nuts: ground amaranth, stone-ground brown rice, stone-ground yellow cornmeal, ground flaxseed meal, ground quinoa, ground sorghum, steel-cut oats, ground almond meal, and ground coconut. These less-processed ingredients, being ground with their fat content, don't enjoy that extended shelf life.

Proper storage allows you the freshest ingredients for the longest period of time. You need to forgo your canister, though.

Flour substitutes should be stored in your refrigerator or freezer. You can keep them in their original packaging with all the nutrition data and other information it provides. Just pop them into a zipper-lock plastic bag or a freezer storage bag to ensure they remain airtight. They'll stay fresh for up to six months. Dating the packages will spare you the unpleasant discovery that the ingredient has gone rancid.

For Good Measure

Although named quick breads, most take about an hour to bake. Quick breads get their name from their fast-fix batters—speedy when compared to the kneading and rising process of yeast breads.

These nutritionally rich alternatives can be paired with healthful fruits, spices, and yogurt. The end results are baked goods packed with protein, fiber, and fat to keep your engine running smoothly, and, of course, keep your blood sugar levels stable.

Mini Cornmeal Muffins

Pick up a small nibble that packs the robust taste of cornmeal. This recipe is gluten-free.

¾ cup fat-free milk

1 TB. fresh lemon juice

1 cup stone-ground yellow cornmeal

½ cup stone-ground brown rice

3 TB. ground flaxseed meal

1 tsp. fine sea salt

½ tsp. baking soda

1 large egg, at room temperature

1 TB. agave nectar

Yield: 2 dozen
Prep time: 15 minutes
Cook time: 10 minutes
Serving size: 2 muffins
Each serving has:
88 calories
2 g fat
0 g saturated fat
16 g carbohydrates
2 g fiber
3 g protein
257 mg sodium

1. Preheat the oven to 400°F. Place a nonstick 24-cup mini muffin pan in the preheating oven.

2. Meanwhile, measure milk, and stir in lemon juice. Let stand to curdle while you prepare the remaining ingredients.

3. In a large bowl, combine yellow cornmeal, stone-ground brown rice, ground flaxseed meal, sea salt, and baking soda. Stir to mix thoroughly.

4. In a small bowl, lightly whisk egg until lemon-colored. Stir in agave nectar to blend. Pour into dry ingredients. Pour in milk mixture. Stir until dry ingredients are moistened.

5. Remove the muffin pan from the preheated oven, and coat with cooking spray.

6. Spoon batter into the muffin cups, filling ¾ full. Bake for 10 minutes or until golden brown. Cool on a wire rack for 5 minutes. Remove muffins to the wire rack to cool. Serve warm, or cool completely.

For Good Measure

Agave nectar offers a lower glycemic index—and is therefore more slowly metabolized—than granulated white sugar.

Pumpkin Pecan Muffins

Spiced pumpkin keeps these muffins tender and moist. This recipe is gluten-free.

Yield: 8 servings
Prep time: 18 minutes
Cook time: 25 minutes
Serving size: 1 muffin
Each serving has:
213 calories
6 g fat
1 g saturated fat
33 g carbohydrates
5 g fiber
6 g protein
169 mg sodium

½ cup ground flaxseed meal

½ cup ground amaranth

¼ cup ground quinoa

¼ cup chopped pecans

½ tsp. xanthan gum

½ tsp. baking soda

¼ tsp. fine sea salt

¾ tsp. ground cinnamon

¼ tsp. ground nutmeg

⅛ tsp. ground cloves

1 large egg, at room temperature

½ cup honey

½ cup canned pure pumpkin

¼ cup fat-free plain yogurt

1. Preheat the oven to 350°F.

2. In a large bowl, combine ground flaxseed meal, ground amaranth, ground quinoa, pecans, xanthan gum, baking soda, sea salt, cinnamon, nutmeg, and cloves. Stir to mix thoroughly.

3. In a medium bowl, whisk egg until lemon-colored. Whisk in honey until well blended. Whisk in pumpkin and yogurt until blended. Add to dry ingredients, and stir until moistened.

4. Spoon batter into 8 muffin cups coated with cooking spray, filling ⅔ full. (Pour a little water into any empty muffin cups.) Bake for 25 minutes or until a cake tester or a wooden toothpick inserted in the center comes out clean.

5. Cool in the muffin cups on a wire rack for 10 minutes. Remove muffins, and cool completely on a wire rack.

For Good Measure

Pouring a little water into any extra cups on your muffin pan will protect the nonstick coating during baking.

Sharp Cheddar Apple Pie Muffins

These dense, single-serving offerings are moist with spiced apples accompanied by an undertone of savory cheddar.

1 cup stone-ground brown rice

⅓ cup ground flaxseed meal

¼ cup steel-cut oats

1 tsp. baking soda

1 tsp. ground cinnamon

½ tsp. ground nutmeg

⅓ cup finely shredded sharp cheddar cheese

1 large egg, at room temperature

⅔ cup fat-free plain yogurt

¼ cup fresh-pressed 100-percent apple juice

2 medium Gala apples, grated (discard cores)

Yield: 9 servings
Prep time: 18 minutes
Cook time: 30 minutes
Serving size: 1 muffin
Each serving has:
161 calories
4 g fat
1 g saturated fat
25 g carbohydrates
3 g fiber
6 g protein
193 mg sodium

1. Preheat the oven to 350°F.

2. In a large bowl, combine stone-ground brown rice, ground flaxseed meal, steel-cut oats, baking soda, cinnamon, and nutmeg. Stir to mix thoroughly. Add cheddar cheese, and stir to distribute evenly.

3. In a medium bowl, whisk egg until lemon-colored. Whisk in yogurt and apple juice. Add grated apples, and stir to blend. Add to dry ingredients, and stir until moistened.

4. Spoon batter into 9 muffin cups coated with cooking spray, filling ¾ full. (Pour a little water into any empty muffin cups.) Bake for 30 minutes or until tops are golden-brown and a cake tester or a wooden toothpick inserted in the center comes out clean. Cool in the muffin cups for 10 minutes on a wire rack. Remove muffins, and cool completely on a wire rack.

 For Good Measure _____

Greek yogurt is strained to produce a thick consistency that supplies more protein with less sugar and sodium than regular yogurt. Creamier fat-free plain yogurt is good for baking. Plus, it supplies about three times the amount of calcium than that found in Greek yogurt.

Blueberry Flax Muffins

Filled with plenty of juicy blueberries, these muffins are sweet and tender. This recipe is gluten-free.

Yield: 7 servings
Prep time: 18 minutes
Cook time: 20 minutes
Serving size: 1 muffin
Each serving has:
245 calories
12 g fat
1 g saturated fat
27 g carbohydrates
7 g fiber
8 g protein
370 mg sodium

1 cup ground flaxseed meal

¾ cup ground almond meal

¼ cup stone-ground brown rice

½ TB. baking soda

¼ tsp. ground cinnamon

¼ tsp. fine sea salt

1 large egg, at room temperature

⅓ cup fat-free plain yogurt

5 TB. agave nectar

1 cup fresh blueberries

1. Preheat the oven to 350°F.

2. In a large bowl, combine ground flaxseed meal, ground almond meal, stone-ground brown rice, baking soda, cinnamon, and sea salt. Stir to mix thoroughly.

3. In a small bowl, whisk egg until lemon-colored. Whisk in yogurt and agave nectar until blended.

4. Stir blueberries into dry ingredients to coat. Add wet ingredients, and stir until moistened.

5. Spoon batter into 7 muffin cups coated with cooking spray, filling ¾ full. (Pour a little water into any empty muffin cups.) Bake for 20 minutes or until browned and a cake tester or a wooden toothpick inserted in the center comes out clean. Cool in the muffin cups on a wire rack for 10 minutes. Remove muffins, and cool completely on the wire rack.

For Good Measure

Ground flaxseed meal can serve as both a grain and a fat replacement in baked goods. To substitute for butter or oil, add three times the amount called for in a recipe—for example, ⅓ cup butter equals 1 cup ground flaxseed meal. Adjust the recipe's liquid, if necessary.

Oatmeal Raisin Muffins

The chewy, steel-cut oats are flecked throughout these brown muffins studded with sweet raisins and spiced with a little cinnamon.

⅔ cup stone-ground brown rice

⅓ cup steel-cut oats

¼ cup ground flaxseed meal

1 tsp. baking soda

½ tsp. ground cinnamon

¼ cup raisins

1 large egg, at room temperature

¼ cup honey

½ cup fat-free plain yogurt

Yield: 6 servings
Prep time: 12 minutes
Cook time: 20 minutes
Serving size: 1 muffin
Each serving has:
215 calories
3 g fat
0 g saturated fat
40 g carbohydrates
4 g fiber
6 g protein
240 mg sodium

1. Preheat the oven to 350°F.

2. In a large bowl, combine stone-ground brown rice, steel-cut oats, ground flaxseed meal, baking soda, and cinnamon. Stir to mix thoroughly. Stir in raisins to coat.

3. In a small bowl, whisk egg until lemon-colored. Whisk in honey until well blended. Whisk in yogurt until blended. Pour into dry ingredients, and stir until moistened.

4. Spoon batter into 6 muffin cups coated with cooking spray. (Pour a little water into any empty muffin cups.) Bake for 20 minutes or until browned and a cake tester or a wooden toothpick inserted in the center comes out clean. Cool in the muffin cups for 5 minutes. Remove muffins, and cool completely on a wire rack.

 No-Flour Power

If you've forgotten to bring your eggs to room temperature, try this trick. Place the eggs in a bowl of warm water for 10 to 15 minutes, just until their shells no longer feel cold.

Peanut Butter in My Chocolate Muffins

These chocolaty treats have a swirl of peanut butter in each bite. This recipe is gluten-free.

Yield: 6 servings
Prep time: 15 to 20 minutes
Cook time: 22 minutes
Serving size: 1 muffin
Each serving has:
251 calories
9 g fat
1 g saturated fat
35 g carbohydrates
4 g fiber
7 g protein
324 mg sodium

½ cup ground almond meal

⅓ cup ground flaxseed meal

⅓ cup ground quinoa

3 TB. natural unsweetened cocoa powder

1 tsp. baking soda

½ tsp. xanthan gum

¼ tsp. fine sea salt

1 large egg, at room temperature

½ cup honey

¼ cup fat-free plain yogurt

1 TB. natural salt-free peanut butter, at room temperature

1. Preheat the oven to 350°F.

2. In a large bowl, combine ground almond meal, ground flaxseed meal, ground quinoa, cocoa powder, baking soda, xanthan gum, and sea salt. Stir to mix thoroughly.

3. In a medium bowl, whisk egg until lemon-colored. Whisk in honey until well blended. Whisk in yogurt until blended. Add to dry ingredients, and stir until moistened.

4. Spoon batter into 6 muffin cups coated with cooking spray, filling ⅔ full. Using the back of the spoon, make a small indentation in the center of each batter-filled cup. Spoon ½ teaspoon peanut butter into each indentation. Using a butter knife, swirl the peanut butter through the batter to produce a marbled effect. (Pour a little water into any empty muffin cups.)

5. Bake for 22 minutes or until a cake tester or a wooden toothpick inserted in the center comes out clean. Cool on a wire rack for 5 to 10 minutes. Remove muffins, and cool completely on the wire rack.

No-Flour Power

Only baking soda is called for in this cookbook's recipes because baking powder includes starch. Baking soda must be exposed to moisture and acid to work. As soon as the wet ingredients come in contact with the dry ingredients, work quickly. Bake as soon as possible to capture the rising.

Double Coconut Muffins

Lightly sweetened, these muffins are chock-full of coconut goodness. This recipe is gluten-free.

½ cup unsweetened medium-cut coconut flakes

6 TB. ground flaxseed meal

¼ cup ground coconut

¼ tsp. baking soda

¼ tsp. fine sea salt

3 large eggs, at room temperature

¼ cup honey

2 TB. fat-free plain yogurt

¼ tsp. vanilla extract

Yield: 6 servings
Prep time: 20 minutes
Cook time: 15 minutes
Serving size: 1 muffin
Each serving has:
237 calories
13 g fat
8 g saturated fat
22 g carbohydrates
6 g fiber
7 g protein
203 mg sodium

1. Preheat the oven to 400°F.

2. In a large bowl, combine coconut flakes, ground flaxseed meal, ground coconut, baking soda, and sea salt. Stir to mix thoroughly.

3. In a medium bowl, whisk eggs until lemon-colored. Whisk in honey until well blended. Whisk in yogurt and vanilla extract until blended. Add to dry ingredients, and stir until moistened.

4. Spoon batter into 6 muffin cups coated with cooking spray, filling half full. (Pour a little water into any empty muffin cups.) Bake for 15 minutes or until a cake tester or a wooden toothpick inserted in the center comes out clean. Cool in the muffin cups for 10 minutes on a wire rack. Remove muffins, and cool completely on the wire rack.

 For Good Measure

Recipes for baked goods call for cooling on a wire rack to allow for even air circulation. Items should be cooled completely before storing in an airtight container or wrapping.

Lip-Puckering Lemon Loaf

This dense, walnut-studded brown bread carries a pleasant lemon flavor—the lemon glaze packs the zing. This recipe is gluten-free.

Yield: 16 servings
Prep time: 25 minutes
Cook time: 50 minutes
Serving size: 1 slice
Each serving has:
185 calories
11 g fat
3 g saturated fat
17 g carbohydrates
2 g fiber
4 g protein
93 mg sodium

3 TB. fresh lemon juice

½ cup fat-free milk

1 cup ground almond meal

½ cup ground amaranth

½ cup chopped walnuts

1 tsp. baking soda

½ tsp. xanthan gum

1 cup plus 2 TB. date sugar

6 TB. unsalted butter, melted

2 large eggs, at room temperature

1 TB. grated lemon zest

1. Preheat the oven to 350°F.

2. Pour 1 tablespoon lemon juice into milk. Set aside to curdle while you prepare the remaining ingredients.

3. In a large bowl, combine ground almond meal, ground amaranth, walnuts, baking soda, and xanthan gum. Stir to mix thoroughly.

4. In a medium bowl, add 1 cup date sugar to melted butter, and stir until moistened. Add eggs and lemon zest, and stir until well blended. Pour in curdled milk, and stir to blend. Add to dry ingredients, and stir until moistened.

5. Pour batter into a 9×5×3 nonstick loaf pan coated with cooking spray, smoothing out top of batter. Bake for 50 minutes or until a cake tester or a wooden toothpick inserted in the center comes out clean.

6. Meanwhile, in a small bowl, combine 2 tablespoons date sugar and 2 tablespoons lemon juice. Stir to blend. When bread is done, spread glaze evenly over top. Cool on a wire rack for 15 minutes before removing bread from the pan to cool completely on the wire rack. Cut into ½-inch slices to serve.

No-Flour Power

When baked goods call for melted butter, it should be cooled before adding to other ingredients. When called for, melt the butter and set it aside to cool to room temperature while you gather the remaining ingredients.

Zesty Zucchini Bread

Nutty and mildly sweet, this bread packs the familiar taste of the ubiquitous summer squash. This recipe is gluten-free.

1 cup finely shredded zucchini	**2 large eggs, at room temperature**
¾ cup ground flaxseed meal	**½ cup honey**
¾ cup ground quinoa	**¼ cup fat-free plain yogurt**
½ cup chopped pecans	**1 tsp. grated lemon zest**
½ tsp. baking soda	**½ tsp. vanilla extract**
½ tsp. fine sea salt	

Yield: 16 servings
Prep time: 25 minutes
Cook time: 60 to 65 minutes
Serving size: 1 slice
Each serving has:
122 calories
5 g fat
0 g saturated fat
16 g carbohydrates
2 g fiber
3 g protein
123 mg sodium

1. Preheat the oven to 350°F.

2. Press shredded zucchini between paper towels to squeeze out moisture.

3. In a large bowl, combine ground flaxseed meal, ground quinoa, pecans, baking soda, and sea salt. Stir to mix thoroughly.

4. In a medium bowl, whisk eggs until lemon-colored. Whisk in honey until well blended. Whisk in yogurt, lemon zest, and vanilla extract until blended. Pour into dry ingredients, and stir just until moistened. Stir in zucchini to distribute evenly.

5. Pour batter into a 9×5×3 nonstick loaf pan coated with cooking spray. Bake for 60 to 65 minutes or until a cake tester or a wooden toothpick inserted in the center comes out clean. Cool on a wire rack for 10 minutes before removing bread from the pan to cool completely on the wire rack. Cut into ½-inch slices to serve.

No-Flour Power _____

Flour substitutes can be measured just as you would flour. Lightly spoon the ground flaxseed meal, ground quinoa, stone-ground yellow cornmeal, or other flour substitutes into a measuring cup; then, level the measurement by scraping off the excess using the back of a butter knife.

Cranberry-Orange Harvest Bread

The orange-sweetened bread offers tart cranberry bits and crunchy pecan nuggets. This recipe is gluten-free.

Yield: 16 servings
Prep time: 18 minutes
Cook time: 1 hour
Serving size: 1 slice
Each serving has:
147 calories
6 g fat
0 g saturated fat
20 g carbohydrates
4 g fiber
4 g protein
119 mg sodium

1 cup ground flaxseed meal

½ cup ground amaranth

½ cup ground sorghum

½ cup chopped pecans

1 tsp. baking soda

½ tsp. xanthan gum

¼ tsp. fine sea salt

1 large egg, at room temperature

½ cup honey

½ cup fresh orange juice

1 tsp. grated orange zest

1 cup coarsely chopped fresh or frozen cranberries

1. Preheat the oven to 350°F.

2. In a large bowl, combine ground flaxseed meal, ground amaranth, ground sorghum, pecans, baking soda, xanthan gum, and sea salt. Stir to mix thoroughly.

3. In a medium bowl, whisk egg until lemon-colored. Whisk in honey until well blended. Whisk in orange juice and orange zest until blended.

4. Stir cranberries into dry ingredients to coat. Stir in orange juice mixture until dry ingredients are moistened. Pour batter into a 9×5×3 nonstick loaf pan, and smooth top.

5. Bake for 1 hour or until a cake tester or a wooden toothpick inserted in the center comes out clean. Cool for 10 minutes on a wire rack before removing bread from the pan to cool completely on the wire rack. Cut into ½-inch slices to serve.

No-Flour Power

Remember that baked goods come together best when the ingredients are at room temperature. If you store your ground whole grains and nuts in the refrigerator or freezer, let them thaw to room temperature before baking.

Banana-Walnut Bread

Hearty enough to stand up to your favorite smears, this bread stands alone with a mild banana flavor accompanied by a nutty crunch. This recipe is gluten-free.

1 cup ground flaxseed meal

1 cup ground quinoa

⅔ cup stone-ground brown rice

½ cup chopped walnuts

1 TB. *xanthan gum*

1 tsp. baking soda

½ tsp. fine sea salt

2 large eggs, at room temperature

½ cup honey

3 very ripe medium bananas, peeled

⅓ cup fat-free plain yogurt

Yield: 16 servings
Prep time: 25 minutes
Cook time: 65 to 70 minutes
Serving size: 1 slice
Each serving has:
188 calories
6 g fat
0 g saturated fat
29 g carbohydrates
4 g fiber
5 g protein
165 mg sodium

1. Preheat the oven to 350°F.

2. In a large bowl, combine ground flaxseed meal, ground quinoa, stone-ground brown rice, walnuts, xanthan gum, baking soda, and sea salt. Stir to mix thoroughly.

3. In a medium bowl, whisk eggs until lemon-colored. Whisk in honey until well blended. Slice in bananas, 1 at a time, mashing mixture with the back of a fork. Whisk in yogurt until blended. Add to dry ingredients, and stir until moistened.

4. Turn batter into a 9×5×3 nonstick loaf pan coated with cooking spray, and smooth out top. Bake for 65 to 70 minutes or until a cake tester or a wooden toothpick inserted in the center comes out clean. Cool on a wire rack for 10 minutes before removing bread from the pan to cool completely on the wire rack. Cut into ½-inch slices to serve.

Words to Digest

Xanthan gum is a polysaccharide that acts as a dietary fiber. It is often used in salad dressings, sauces, and ice creams. In addition, it can be used in gluten-free recipes because of its ability to act as a binder.

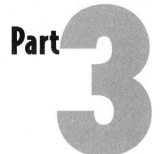

Part 3

Lunches and Lighter Fare

Whether an everyday midday meal, a family-and-friends gathering, or a nosh-nibbling party, you'll find plenty of flour-full foods. You don't want to be the one not having fun.

So celebrate the great flour-free ingredients that allow you to enjoy delicious sandwiches, soups, salads, and appetizers aplenty. With a little creativity, great recipes, and a well-stocked kitchen, others will be eyeing up your favorite foods.

Chapter 8

Sandwich Switcheroo

In This Chapter

- ◆ Flourless bread substitutes for tasty sandwich selections
- ◆ Creative, edible vehicles as sandwich bread stand-ins
- ◆ Standalone sandwiches

A sandwich really isn't a sandwich without the bread. And bread really isn't bread without flour, right?

Maybe not. With the help of some food companies and a little ingenuity on your part, lunch can still be a scrumptious sandwich.

Think Outside the Bread Box

You can find breads that fit your flour-free eating plan. A number of food producers offer flourless breads in any number of forms: regular loaves, cinnamon-raisin loaves, buns, pitas, tortillas, and English muffins. For those who need to avoid gluten, you can use wheat-free breads. Look for breads that contain less sugar and more fiber. Check out Appendix C for resources.

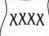

No-Flour Power _____

If your sprouted-grain bread is frozen, thaw the slices you need by removing them to a plastic zipper-lock bag placed in the refrigerator. Or put frozen slices directly into a toaster. Microwaves aren't good for thawing breads, as they leave them dried out.

Because sprouted-grain breads are made with whole grains and contain no preservatives, you'll often find them in the freezer case. Some grocers keep them on their shelves, so you'll want to check there, too. For the greatest freshness, you should store sprouted-grain breads in your refrigerator or freezer.

Packed with valuable nutrients, bread becomes more than what holds your sandwich together. Of course, not all sandwiches need bread for serving. Why not get creative? Lettuce wraps, avocado boats, and simply bunless can be just the beginning of your sandwich switcheroos.

Fold-Over Corn Tortillas

While warm, these thick and hearty cornmeal-and-brown-rice-based tortillas can be folded in half as a flatbread. This recipe is gluten-free.

1 cup stone-ground yellow cornmeal

½ cup stone-ground brown rice

1 tsp. xanthan gum

½ tsp. fine sea salt

¾ cup warm water (110°F)

Yield: 6 tortillas
Prep time: 8 minutes
Cook time: 24 minutes
Serving size: 1 tortilla
Each serving has:
126 calories
1 g fat
0 g saturated fat
26 g carbohydrates
3 g fiber
3 g protein
198 mg sodium

1. In a medium bowl, stir together yellow cornmeal, stone-ground brown rice, xanthan gum, and sea salt. Pour in ½ cup warm water, and stir well to moisten dry ingredients.

2. Add remaining ¼ cup warm water, and stir, pulling dough into a ball, cleaning the side of the bowl. Divide dough into 6 equal portions.

3. Lightly dust the work surface, a rolling pin, and your hands with additional stone-ground brown rice. Turn 1 dough portion over on work surface to coat with stone-ground brown rice. Roll into a ball, working gently with dough. Gently flatten ball into a 3- to 4-inch circle, pushing edges back in as they crack. Gently roll into a 6- to 7-inch circle.

4. Heat a 9-inch nonstick skillet over medium heat. When hot, coat with cooking spray. With a large 4-inch spatula, carefully loosen dough from the work surface, and transfer to the skillet. Cook for 2 minutes or until top of tortilla begins to puff slightly and underside is browned.

5. With the spatula, lift tortilla, and coat the skillet with cooking spray again. Turn tortilla, and cook for 2 minutes or until the underside is browned. Remove from the skillet to cool.

6. While tortilla cooks, repeat rolling-out process with remaining dough portions. Cook each as directed, and serve warm or cool. Store in an airtight container in the refrigerator if not serving the same day.

For Good Measure

Xanthan gum can be used as a gluten replacement, giving your breads made without wheat flours a little elasticity.

Fish Soft Tacos

Hot and cold, spicy and creamy are folded into a soft corn shell. This recipe is gluten-free.

Yield: 3 servings
Prep time: 5 minutes
Cook time: 8 minutes
Serving size: 1 taco
Each serving has:
284 calories
11 g fat
3 g saturated fat
30 g carbohydrates
3 g fiber
18 g protein
491 mg sodium

1 TB. Taco Seasoning Blend (see Chapter 13)

1 (10-oz.) fillet skinless fresh catfish

2 tsp. fresh lime juice

3 prepared Fold-Over Corn Tortillas (recipe earlier in this chapter)

½ cup shredded romaine lettuce

⅓ cup finely diced tomatoes

3 TB. reduced-fat sour cream

1 medium jalapeño pepper, seeded (optional) and sliced

1. Heat a large nonstick skillet over medium heat. When hot, coat with cooking spray.

2. Rub Taco Seasoning Blend on both sides of catfish. Cook for 4 minutes on each side or until opaque and fish flakes easily with a fork.

3. Remove the skillet from heat. Drizzle lime juice over catfish. Cut catfish into smaller pieces.

4. Divide catfish among Fold-Over Corn Tortillas, arranging down the centers. Top fish with lettuce, tomatoes, sour cream, and jalapeño pepper slices. Fold tortillas around filling to serve.

Starch Guard

Remember to read ingredient lists. Fat-free sour creams are typically bulked up with starches and sugars. Check the reduced-fat sour cream labels for the same. Starch-free, sugar-free, reduced-fat sour creams are available.

Tortilla Crust Personal Pizza

Enjoy the traditional taste of Italian-style tomato sauce and melted cheese on a thin crust without a call to the local pizza parlor. This recipe is gluten-free.

1½ TB. tomato paste

1 TB. water

½ tsp. chopped fresh basil

½ tsp. chopped fresh oregano

⅛ tsp. garlic powder

⅛ tsp. onion powder

1 prepared Fold-Over Corn Tortilla (recipe earlier in this chapter)

3 TB. shredded low-moisture, part-skim mozzarella cheese

1 TB. shredded Parmesan cheese

Yield: 1 serving
Prep time: 3 minutes
Cook time: 5 minutes
Serving size: 1 pizza
Each serving has:
244 calories
7 g fat
4 g saturated fat
33 g carbohydrates
4 g fiber
13 g protein
608 mg sodium

1. Preheat the oven to 350°F.

2. In a small bowl, combine tomato paste and water, and stir to blend. Stir in basil, oregano, garlic powder, and onion powder.

3. Spoon tomato paste mixture onto prepared Fold-Over Corn Tortilla, spreading sauce evenly over tortilla and leaving a small margin at the edge.

4. Sprinkle mozzarella cheese and Parmesan cheese over sauce. Bake on a small nonstick baking sheet for 5 minutes or until cheeses are melted. Cut into 4 slices to serve.

Variation: Top the pizza with your favorite toppings before baking. Try a sprinkling of chopped green peppers, chopped onions, sliced mushrooms, diced tomatoes, sliced black olives, or any of your personal favorites.

 For Good Measure

Tomato paste can be a single-ingredient product easily blended into a savory pizza sauce with your own herbs and spices. However, some tomato pastes and canned tomato sauces may include sugar, salt, and those mysterious "natural flavorings." Be sure to read the labels.

Turkey Dijon Lettuce Wrap

Crisp apple slices sweeten up the smooth meat and cheese wrapped in equally crisp lettuce. There is no bread, so the taste doesn't get lost. This recipe is gluten-free.

Yield: 1 serving
Prep time: 3 minutes
Serving size: 1 sandwich
Each serving has:
148 calories
5 g fat
3 g saturated fat
10 g carbohydrates
2 g fiber
15 g protein
447 mg sodium

4 large leaves red leaf lettuce

1 thin slice reduced-fat Swiss cheese

1 tsp. Dijon mustard

2 slices natural deli turkey breast

¼ medium Gala apple, cored and very thinly sliced

1. Remove the lower portions of lettuce leaves with thick stems. (Reserve for another use.) Arrange the leafy portions of lettuce leaves vertically on a plate, overlapping to make slightly larger than the size of turkey slices.

2. Arrange cheese slice in the center of lettuce leaves. Spread half of Dijon mustard over cheese. Layer turkey breast slices on top, and spread remaining Dijon mustard over turkey. Arrange apple slices on top vertically.

3. Roll sandwich into lettuce leaves horizontally, rolling as tightly as possible to enclose filling. Serve immediately.

 For Good Measure

You can save on the unnecessary additives found in traditional deli options by choosing natural turkey breast when buying deli meat.

Asian Chicken Salad on Toasted Sprouted-Grain Bread

With the added crunch of snow peas, this oil-and-vinegar–based chicken salad is mildly spicy and flavored with sesame seed oil.

½ cup finely chopped cooked chicken breast

2 TB. finely chopped snow peas

1 TB. unseasoned rice vinegar

2 tsp. extra-virgin olive oil

1 tsp. sesame seed oil

¼ tsp. chili powder

⅛ tsp. ground ginger

⅛ tsp. fine sea salt

⅛ tsp. freshly ground black pepper

2 slices sprouted-grain bread, toasted

Yield: 1 serving
Prep time: 5 minutes
Chill time: 30 minutes
Serving size: 1 sandwich
Each serving has:
407 calories
18 g fat
3 g saturated fat
32 g carbohydrates
7 g fiber
30 g protein
488 mg sodium

1. In a small bowl, combine chicken breast, snow peas, rice vinegar, extra-virgin olive oil, sesame seed oil, chili powder, ginger, sea salt, and black pepper. Stir to coat evenly. Cover and chill for at least 30 minutes to allow flavors to meld.

2. Stir chicken mixture again before serving. Spoon onto 1 bread slice, spreading out evenly. Close sandwich firmly with remaining bread slice. Cut in half to serve, if desired. Serve immediately.

No-Flour Power

If you're using leftover chicken that was seasoned with sea salt and black pepper when prepared, you may want to omit these ingredients from the chicken salad.

To prepare fresh snow peas, snap off the ends and pull down the length of the snow pea to remove the thick string that may grow along the "seam."

Tuna Avocado Baby Swiss Melts

This melted Baby Swiss and creamy avocado boat allows you to enjoy the pleasantly crunchy tuna salad out-of-hand with a napkin at hand. This recipe is gluten-free.

Yield: 2 servings
Prep time: 10 minutes
Cook time: 3 minutes
Serving size: 1 melt
Each serving has:
310 calories
24 g fat
7 g saturated fat
7 g carbohydrates
4 g fiber
16 g protein
293 mg sodium

1 (2.6-oz.) pkg. light tuna packed in water

2 TB. finely chopped celery

2 TB. Really Ranch Dressing (see Chapter 10)

1 medium ripe, slightly firm avocado

2 thin slices Baby Swiss cheese

1. Preheat the oven to 350°F.

2. In a small bowl, combine tuna, celery, and Really Ranch Dressing. Stir to coat evenly.

3. Cut avocado in half lengthwise, twisting halves to separate. Push a knife blade slightly into the pit, and twist to remove. Run the bowl of a spoon between the peel and the flesh of the avocado to remove avocado halves. Cut a slice off the bottom of each avocado half to allow it to sit flat, taking care not to cut open the hollow.

4. Place avocado halves on a small nonstick baking sheet. Spoon half of tuna mixture over each avocado half, pushing into the hollow and spreading over the top of the avocado half. Cover each with 1 cheese slice. Bake for 3 minutes or until cheese is melted. Serve immediately.

No-Flour Power

XXXX

If you need to speed the ripening of an avocado, place the avocado in a brown paper bag with a tomato, apple, banana, or other ethylene-gas-producing fruit.

Mediterranean Vegetable Crepes

The region's most popular veggies—roasted red peppers, spinach, and olives—offer their bold flavors in the skillet-sizzled filling for this savory crepe sandwich you can share with a friend. This recipe is gluten-free.

1 tsp. extra-virgin olive oil

½ cup thinly sliced red onions

1 medium clove garlic, minced

1 cup packed spinach leaves

Pinch fine sea salt

Pinch freshly ground black pepper

¼ cup water-packed roasted red peppers, drained

4 medium kalamata olives, drained and chopped

¼ cup shredded brick or Monterey Jack cheese

1 (8-inch) prepared Basic Crepe Batter (see Chapter 6) crepe

Yield: 2 servings
Prep time: 2 minutes
Cook time: 5 minutes
Serving size: 1 crepe
Each serving has:
269 calories
18 g fat
5 g saturated fat
17 g carbohydrates
2 g fiber
10 g protein
522 mg sodium

1. Heat a 9-inch nonstick skillet over medium heat. When hot, add extra-virgin olive oil. Stir in red onions. Cook and stir for 2 minutes or until red onions are softened.

2. Stir in garlic, and cook for 1 minute.

3. Add spinach, sea salt, and black pepper. Cook and stir for 1 minute or until spinach is wilted.

4. Add roasted red peppers and olives. Cook and stir for 1 minute or until heated through.

5. Remove the skillet from the heat. Add cheese, and stir to distribute as it melts.

6. Turn out mixture onto one half of prepared crepe. Fold the other half over top. Cut in half, and serve hot.

For Good Measure

When measuring loose, voluminous ingredients such as leafy greens, the term "packed" indicates that the ingredient should be pushed tightly into the measuring cup for the most accurate amount.

Broiled Portobello Mushroom Burger

This fork-and-knife sandwich lets you savor the meaty mushroom cap topped with sweet red peppers, sautéd red onions, and provolone cheese without the soggy bun. This recipe is gluten-free.

Yield: 1 serving
Prep time: 3 minutes
Cook time: 14 minutes
Serving size: 1 burger
Each serving has:
150 calories
9 g fat
3 g saturated fat
10 g carbohydrates
2 g fiber
8 g protein
527 mg sodium

1 medium portobello mushroom cap

1 tsp. extra-virgin olive oil

1 (¼-inch) slice red onion

¼ cup water-packed roasted red peppers, drained

Pinch fine sea salt

Pinch freshly ground black pepper

1 thin slice, reduced-fat provolone cheese

1. Preheat the broiler to high.

2. Remove stem from portobello mushroom cap and discard. Place mushroom cap gill side down on a broiler pan coated with cooking spray. Broil 6 inches from heat for 8 minutes or until softened and browned.

3. Meanwhile, heat a small skillet over medium-low heat. When hot, add extra-virgin olive oil. Separate red onion slice into rings, and add to the skillet. Cook, stirring frequently, for 3 to 5 minutes or until tender.

4. Turn off heat under the skillet. Add roasted red peppers, sea salt, and black pepper to red onion mixture. Stir to mix.

5. Turn mushroom cap gill side up on the broiler pan, and fill with red onion mixture. Broil for 5 minutes or until mushroom cap is tender. Arrange cheese slice over filling. Broil for 1 minute or just until cheese begins to bubble and brown. Serve hot.

Starch Guard

Be certain to position the oven rack to broil 6 inches from the heating element. Extra-virgin olive oil has a relatively low smoke point and can start to smoke if too close to the high heat.

Broiled Black Bean Burgers

Crispy outside, "juicy" inside, these veggie burgers offer a hint of Southwest flavor with the addition of cumin and cilantro. This recipe is gluten-free.

2 tsp. extra-virgin olive oil

¾ cup diced yellow onions

2 cups finely chopped white button mushrooms

2 medium cloves garlic, minced

¼ tsp. ground cumin

1 cup cooked black beans

¼ cup chopped fresh cilantro

1¾ cups sprouted-grain breadcrumbs

¼ tsp. fine sea salt

¼ tsp. freshly ground black pepper

Yield: 4 servings
Prep time: 5 minutes
Cook time: 20 minutes
Serving size: 1 burger
Each serving has:
150 calories
3 g fat
0 g saturated fat
24 g carbohydrates
6 g fiber
7 g protein
188 mg sodium

1. Preheat the broiler on high.

2. Heat a large skillet over medium heat. When hot, add extra-virgin olive oil. Add onions and cook, stirring frequently, for 5 minutes or until translucent.

3. Add mushrooms, garlic, and cumin. Cook, stirring occasionally, for 5 minutes or until liquid is released from mushrooms.

4. In a food processor, combine mushroom mixture, black beans, and cilantro. Process on high speed for 20 seconds or until mixed. Stop to scrape down sides as necessary.

5. In a large bowl, combine black bean mixture, breadcrumbs, sea salt, and black pepper. Stir to mix. Shape into 4 (3½-inch) patties.

6. Arrange patties on a broiler pan coated with cooking spray. Broil 6 inches from the heating element for 5 minutes or until browned. Turn patties over and broil for 5 minutes until browned and crisped. Serve plain or on flourless sandwich buns with your favorite burger fixings.

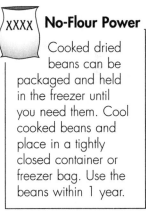

No-Flour Power

Cooked dried beans can be packaged and held in the freezer until you need them. Cool cooked beans and place in a tightly closed container or freezer bag. Use the beans within 1 year.

Chapter 9

Kettle Kreations

In This Chapter

- Satisfying soups with flour-free pasta alternatives
- Comforting soups and stews thickened with flour substitutes
- Flourless ingredients that naturally enhance the body of simmered soups and stews

A bowl of body-warming soup or stew is comfort food at its best. You love it piping hot with a satisfying consistency. Of course, you don't want starchy thickeners swimming in your soup, ruining your more healthful eating plan. Hold on to your soup spoon! Alternative thickeners won't leave you flat.

In the Thick of It

Open your pantry and you'll likely find an array of traditional thickeners that are often loaded with empty carbohydrates—all-purpose flour, cornstarch, arrowroot, potato flakes, and tapioca. You'd like to eliminate these ingredients from your diet, but you're lamenting the runny, lifeless recipes that foreshadow.

You needn't fear soupy stews, thin sauces, and droopy puddings. Go ahead and toss the starchy set. Soups and stews, sauces and gravies, and puddings and other desserts will stand up to the challenge with some simple substitutions. Whether sweet or savory dishes, a new take on thickening agents will keep your recipes from running away on you. Flour-free thickeners like eggs, butter, cream, tomato paste, vegetable purées, stone-ground brown rice, unflavored gelatin, and simple reduction will allow you to have your soup and eat it, too.

XXXX **No-Flour Power**

Some soups can be thickened by puréeing a portion of the soup in a blender before stirring it back into the soup.

Home-Style Chicken Noodle Soup

Filled with chicken, veggies, and brown-rice noodles, this home-prepared soup tastes deliciously fresh while keeping the sodium levels in check. This recipe can be gluten-free if the chicken broth you use is gluten-free.

6 cups fat-free, reduced-sodium chicken broth

1½ cups ½-inch cubed cooked chicken breast

¾ cup finely chopped carrots

¾ cup diced yellow onions

½ cup sliced celery

1 medium clove garlic, minced

3 TB. chopped fresh parsley

¼ tsp. fine sea salt

¼ tsp. freshly ground black pepper

2 cups broken 2-inch pieces brown rice fettuccini pasta

Yield: 7 servings
Prep time: 3 minutes
Cook time: 27 minutes
Serving size: 1 cup
Each serving has:
156 calories
2 g fat
1 g saturated fat
22 g carbohydrates
2 g fiber
13 g protein
510 mg sodium

1. In a large saucepan, combine chicken broth, chicken, carrots, onions, celery, garlic, parsley, sea salt, and black pepper. Stir. Bring to a boil over high heat. Reduce heat to medium-low, and simmer for 5 minutes.

2. Gradually stir in broken pasta. *Simmer* for 15 minutes or until pasta and vegetables are tender, stirring occasionally to keep pasta from sticking. Serve hot.

Words to Digest

Simmer is a stage where the cooking liquid barely bubbles, boiling gently.

Italian Vegetable Minestrone

Chock-full of tender vegetables, fresh herbs, and hearty beans, a bowlful of this classic Italian soup will warm you up and fill you up. This recipe is gluten-free.

Yield: 7 servings
Prep time: 3 minutes
Cook time: 38 minutes
Serving size: 1 cup
Each serving has:
149 calories
1 g fat
0 g saturated fat
28 g carbohydrates
6 g fiber
6 g protein
521 mg sodium

4 cups fat-free, reduced-sodium vegetable broth

1 (14.5-oz.) can petite-cut diced tomatoes, undrained

1½ cups shredded green cabbage

½ cup diced yellow onions

¼ cup thinly sliced celery

¼ cup finely chopped carrots

1 medium clove garlic, minced

1 cup cooked garbanzo beans

1 cup cooked light red kidney beans

1 cup thinly sliced, halved zucchini

1 cup packed fresh spinach

1 cup brown rice shells pasta

3 TB. chopped fresh basil

2 TB. chopped fresh oregano

¼ tsp. fine sea salt

¼ tsp. freshly ground black pepper

1. In a soup pot, combine vegetable broth, tomatoes, cabbage, onions, celery, carrots, garlic, garbanzo beans, and kidney beans. Bring to a boil over high heat. Reduce heat to medium-low. Simmer, stirring occasionally, for 15 minutes.

2. Add zucchini, spinach, pasta, basil, oregano, sea salt, and black pepper. Stir. Return to a simmer, and simmer for 15 minutes or until vegetables and pasta are tender.

No-Flour Power _____

Prepared broths may contain a varying degree of sugars, starches, and other additives. Read labels to make the best buys. Of course, if you prepare your own stocks at home, you can control exactly what goes into them.

Chinese Hot and Sour Soup

Pleasantly sour with a touch of heat, the chicken broth boasts plenty of mushrooms with bits of spicy garlic and ginger along with strips of subtle green onions and bamboo shoots. This recipe can be gluten-free if the chicken broth is gluten-free.

½ oz. dried shiitake mushrooms

1¼ cups boiling water

3 cups fat-free, reduced-sodium chicken broth

¼ cup unseasoned rice vinegar

2½ TB. naturally brewed soy sauce

2 medium green onions, finely julienned

2 TB. finely julienned bamboo shoots

2 medium cloves garlic, minced

½ TB. minced peeled fresh ginger

1 cup fat-free, reduced-sodium chicken broth, chilled

¼ tsp. hot chili oil, or more to taste

2 TB. stone-ground brown rice

1½ cups thinly slivered white button mushrooms

4 oz. firm tofu, cut into ¼-inch cubes

¼ tsp. fine sea salt

Yield: 5 servings
Prep time: 1 hour 5 minutes
Cook time: 16 minutes
Serving size: 1 cup
Each serving has:
82 calories
2 g fat
0 g saturated fat
9 g carbohydrates
2 g fiber
7 g protein
937 mg sodium

1. In a small bowl, soak shiitake mushrooms in boiling water for 1 hour or until rehydrated. Drain. Remove stems, and thinly sliver mushrooms.

2. In a large saucepan, combine 3 cups chicken broth, rice vinegar, and soy sauce. Bring to a boil over high heat. Add shiitake mushrooms, green onions, bamboo shoots, garlic, and ginger. Stir. Return to a boil. Reduce heat to medium-low, and simmer for 8 minutes.

3. Meanwhile, combine 1 cup chilled chicken broth and hot chili oil. Place stone-ground brown rice in a container with a tight-fitting lid. Add hot chili oil mixture. Cover and shake until well blended. Slowly stir mixture into the saucepan. Add button mushrooms, tofu, and sea salt. Return to a simmer, and simmer for 2 minutes or until slightly thickened. Serve hot.

Starch Guard

Read the ingredients lists on the naturally brewed soy sauce options. Even some naturally brewed varieties may include sugars and other unwanted additions.

Savory Oatmeal Soup

This hearty, whole-grain soup is packed with carrots, mushrooms, and broccoli for a flavorful twist on steel-cut oats.

Yield: 4 servings
Prep time: 3 minutes
Cook time: 27 minutes
Serving size: ¾ cup
Each serving has:
112 calories
3 g fat
1 g saturated fat
17 g carbohydrates
3 g fiber
5 g protein
494 mg sodium

1 tsp. extra-virgin olive oil

¼ cup diced yellow onions

¼ cup sliced celery

¼ cup finely chopped carrots

½ cup sliced white button mushrooms

1 medium clove garlic, minced

3 cups fat-free, reduced-sodium chicken broth

½ cup steel-cut oats

¼ tsp. fine sea salt

¼ tsp. fresh ground black pepper

1 cup chopped fresh broccoli

1. Heat a large saucepan over medium heat. When hot, add extra-virgin olive oil. Add onions, celery, carrots, mushrooms, and garlic. Cook and stir for 5 minutes or until vegetables are softened and golden brown.

2. Gradually pour in chicken broth. Add steel-cut oats, sea salt, and black pepper. Stir. Bring to a boil over high heat.

3. Reduce heat to low. Cover and simmer for 10 minutes, stirring occasionally. Stir in broccoli. Cover and simmer, stirring occasionally, for 10 more minutes or until oats and broccoli are tender. Serve hot.

For Good Measure

Fat-free, reduced-sodium chicken broth can be replaced by fat-free, reduced-sodium vegetable broth to make any meatless soup, stew, or gravy a vegetarian dish.

Quick-Fix Mac and White Bean Stoup

This thick soup—or thin stew—enjoys the heartiness of quinoa macaroni pasta and great Northern beans in a vegetable-enhanced broth. This recipe can be gluten-free if the chicken broth is gluten-free.

2 cups cooked great Northern beans

2 cups fat-free, reduced-sodium chicken broth

1 cup peeled, diced tomatoes

¾ cup uncooked quinoa elbow macaroni pasta

¼ cup finely chopped green bell peppers

¼ cup diced yellow onions

1 medium clove garlic, minced

1 TB. chopped fresh basil

¼ tsp. fine sea salt

¼ tsp. freshly ground black pepper

Yield: 4 servings
Prep time: 2 minutes
Cook time: 18 minutes
Serving size: 1 cup
Each serving has:
195 calories
1 g fat
0 g saturated fat
37 g carbohydrates
8 g fiber
10 g protein
371 mg sodium

1. In a large saucepan, combine beans, chicken broth, tomatoes, pasta, green bell peppers, onions, garlic, basil, sea salt, and black pepper. Bring to a boil over high heat, stirring occasionally to keep pasta from sticking.

2. Reduce heat to low. Cover and simmer, stirring occasionally, for 15 minutes or until pasta and vegetables are tender. Serve hot.

Variation: Substitute a 15¼-ounce can great Northern beans, rinsed and drained, for the cooked beans.

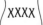 **No-Flour Power** _____

To peel a tomato easily, cut an X in the blossom end. Dunk the tomato in boiling water for 20 seconds. Remove and, with the tip of a sharp knife, peel off the skin.

Rib-Sticking Beef Stew

Tender beef cubes and chunky vegetables pack the seasoned beef broth thickened with stone-ground brown rice instead of flour. This recipe is gluten-free.

Yield: 6 servings
Prep time: 5 minutes
Cook time: 2 hours 35 minutes
Serving size: 1 cup
Each serving has:
174 calories
4 g fat
1 g saturated fat
16 g carbohydrates
3 g fiber
19 g protein
940 mg sodium

1 lb. cubed stew beef, well-trimmed	1 medium green bell pepper, seeded, ribs removed, and chopped
3 cups fat-free, reduced-sodium beef broth	1 medium yellow onion, chopped
¼ tsp. plus ½ TB. fine sea salt	1 medium rib celery, sliced
⅛ tsp. freshly ground black pepper	1 cup small button mushrooms, stems trimmed
3 medium carrots, peeled and coarsely chopped	1 bay leaf
1 medium sweet potato, ends trimmed and coarsely chopped	½ cup cold water
	2 TB. stone-ground brown rice

For Good Measure

Sweet potatoes, while not truly yams (a completely different tuber), may be labeled as such in your local supermarket. Whether yellow-skinned with yellow flesh or dark-red-skinned with orange flesh, these are sweet potatoes—even if the label reads "yams."

1. In a soup pot over medium heat, cook stew beef for 7 minutes, turning to brown all sides. Drain well.

2. Return the saucepan to the heat. Add beef broth, ¼ teaspoon sea salt, and black pepper, and stir. Bring to a boil over high heat. Reduce heat to low. Cover and simmer for 2 hours or until beef is tender.

3. Add carrots, sweet potato, green bell pepper, onion, celery, mushrooms, and bay leaf. Stir in ½ tablespoon sea salt. Return to a boil over high heat. Reduce heat to low. Cover and simmer for 30 minutes or until vegetables are tender.

4. In a small container with a tight-fitting lid, pour cold water into stone-ground brown rice. Cover and shake until blended. Pour into stew and stir. Return to a boil over high heat, and stir until stew begins to thicken. Remove from heat. Remove bay leaf before serving. Serve hot.

Cajun Shrimp Stew with Browned Flourless Roux

A thick, tasty brown roux coats small pink shrimp simply and deliciously. This recipe is gluten-free.

2 TB. unsalted butter

3 TB. stone-ground brown rice

⅛ tsp. fine sea salt

⅛ tsp. freshly ground black pepper

1 cup finely chopped green bell peppers

½ cup diced yellow onions

⅓ cup sliced celery

3 medium cloves garlic, minced

1 TB. tomato paste

1 cup water

1 (14-oz.) pkg. peeled, deveined, tail-off, cooked, small frozen shrimp

Yield: 4 servings
Prep time: 3 minutes
Cook time: 1 hour
Serving size: 1 cup
Each serving has:
199 calories
7 g fat
4 g saturated fat
12 g carbohydrates
2 g fiber
21 g protein
635 mg sodium

1. In a large saucepan over medium heat, melt butter until bubbly. Whisk in stone-ground brown rice, sea salt, and black pepper. Cook, whisking constantly, for 3 minutes or until roux is a deep golden brown.

2. Reduce heat to low. Stir in green bell peppers, onions, celery, and garlic. Cover and cook for 10 minutes.

3. Stir in tomato paste and water. Return to a boil over high heat. Reduce heat to low. Cover and simmer for 30 minutes.

4. Stir in shrimp. Cover and cook over low heat for 10 minutes or until shrimp is heated through. Serve over cooked long-grain brown rice, if desired.

 For Good Measure

A roux is traditionally made from flour mixed with a fat, such as butter, that's cooked before adding a liquid. Stone-ground brown rice is a good alternative for the flour because of its thickening properties.

Chapter 10

More Wholesome Salads and Dressings

In This Chapter

- ◆ Fresh-tasting salad dressings with simple ingredients
- ◆ Flour-free, added-sugar-free salad options
- ◆ Tasty salad toppers to enliven green salads

When you're hungry for something crisp and fresh, a salad can hit the spot. Whether a simple green salad tossed with your favorite veggies and toppings, a prepared pasta salad, or a fruit salad, your mouth can't help but delight in the mix of textures and decadent dressings.

The High Price of Convenience Foods

It seems so simple. You pick up a bottle of salad dressing at the supermarket and pop it in the fridge. Now, anytime you make a salad, the bottled dressing is ready to go—along with its sugars, starches, additives, and preservatives. Most likely, ever since you started reading food labels more carefully, you're less sure of the convenience factor.

If it's convenience you crave, nothing is more convenient than preparing the salad dressings you want when you want them. Preparation is quick and easy. Ingredients are fresh and flavorful. Plus, you know exactly what you're pouring over your salads.

Grab your whisk or blender and whip up a fresh-made salad dressing. Your family and friends will be impressed. Only you will know how simple it is.

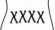

No-Flour Power

If your whisk is dirty or maybe you just don't have one, grab a small fork instead, using the same whisking wrist action. Or the ingredients for a liquid salad dressing can be combined in a jar with a tight-fitting lid. Shake well to blend.

Honey-Mustard Vinaigrette

Pleasantly sweet and sour, this golden dressing perks up your favorite greens and salad vegetables. This recipe is gluten-free.

2 TB. extra-virgin olive oil

4 tsp. prepared yellow mustard

4 tsp. honey

2 tsp. red wine vinegar

⅛ tsp. garlic powder

⅛ tsp. fine sea salt

Yield: 5 servings
Prep time: 1 minute
Serving size: 1 tablespoon
Each serving has:
67 calories
5 g fat
1 g saturated fat
5 g carbohydrates
0 g fiber
0 g protein
100 mg sodium

1. In a small bowl, combine extra-virgin olive oil, yellow mustard, honey, red wine vinegar, garlic powder, and sea salt. Whisk until well blended. Serve immediately.

2. Cover and refrigerate any leftovers, whisking again before serving.

 For Good Measure

Honey should only be enjoyed by those over one year of age. Infants' digestive systems may be unable to process bacterial spores that can be found in honey.

Herb-Flecked Italian Dressing

Nicely seasoned with a pleasant lemon undertone, this dressing enjoys the bright flavor of fresh-made dressing. This recipe is gluten-free.

Yield: 28 servings
Prep time: 2 minutes
Chill time: 1 hour
Serving size: 1 tablespoon
Each serving has:
93 calories
10 g fat
2 g saturated fat
1 g carbohydrates
0 g fiber
0 g protein
20 mg sodium

1⅓ cups extra-virgin olive oil

¼ cup red wine vinegar

¼ cup fresh lemon juice

2 tsp. agave nectar

2 medium cloves garlic, *minced*

½ tsp. dried basil

½ tsp. dried oregano

¼ tsp. fine sea salt

¼ tsp. freshly ground black pepper

1. In a 2-cup or larger measuring cup, measure extra-virgin olive oil. Add red wine vinegar, lemon juice, agave nectar, garlic, basil, oregano, sea salt, and black pepper. Whisk until blended. Transfer to a serving cruet, if desired.

2. Cover and chill for at least 1 hour before serving. Whisk or shake to blend again before serving.

Words to Digest

Minced instructs cooks to cut an ingredient into very small pieces, even smaller than diced. Minced foods should be ⅛-inch pieces or smaller. Garlic should be cut as small as you can make it.

Really Ranch Dressing

Flecked with green herbs, this creamy dressing is seasoned with traditional ranch flavors in tangy sour cream.

¼ cup Fresh-Made Mayonnaise (recipe later in this chapter)

¼ cup reduced-fat sour cream

½ tsp. dried chives

¼ tsp. dried dill weed

¼ tsp. garlic powder

¼ tsp. onion powder

¼ tsp. fine sea salt

⅛ tsp. freshly ground black pepper

Yield: 8 servings
Prep time: 2 minutes
Chill time: 30 minutes
Serving size: 1 tablespoon
Each serving has:
67 calories
7 g fat
2 g saturated fat
1 g carbohydrates
0 g fiber
1 g protein
88 mg sodium

1. In a small bowl, combine Fresh-Made Mayonnaise, sour cream, chives, dill weed, garlic powder, onion powder, sea salt, and black pepper. Stir to blend.

2. Cover and chill for at least 30 minutes before serving. Stir to blend again before serving. Use within 5 days.

For Good Measure

Recipes provide a guide for creating delectable foods. When trying a new recipe, prepare it as given, and then adjust the seasoning to your personal taste. Have fun!

Fresh-Made Mayonnaise

Preparing this homemade mayonnaise with extra-virgin olive oil gives it a distinctly olive-infused flavor. If you prefer a milder taste, you can use canola oil instead. This recipe is gluten-free.

Yield: 10 servings
Prep time: 8 minutes
Serving size: 1 tablespoon
Each serving has:
113 calories
12 g fat
2 g saturated fat
0 g carbohydrates
0 g fiber
1 g protein
30 mg sodium

2 large pasteurized egg yolks

½ cup extra-virgin olive oil or canola oil

Pinch fine sea salt

Pinch freshly ground black pepper

2 TB. red wine vinegar

1. Place egg yolks in a blender. Cover and blend on the lowest speed for 20 seconds or until lemon-colored.

2. Remove the cap from the blender's lid, and hold it ajar over the opening. With the blender running, very slowly add extra-virgin olive oil, drop by drop, for 30 seconds.

3. With the blender running, add remaining extra-virgin olive oil in a very fine stream. (This should take about 4 minutes.)

4. Stop the blender. (Mixture should be creamy.) Add sea salt and black pepper to the mixture. Pour in 1 tablespoon red wine vinegar. Blend on the lowest speed for 5 seconds.

5. Transfer mayonnaise to a small bowl with a tight-fitting lid. Whisk in remaining 1 tablespoon red wine vinegar to taste. Cover and refrigerate for up to 5 days.

Starch Guard

Always opt for pasteurized eggs when preparing uncooked and undercooked egg dishes. Regular eggs can be contaminated with salmonella bacteria, which can cause sickness or even death. Look for eggs marked as pasteurized next to regular eggs in your grocer's refrigerator case.

Cool-and-Crisp Waldorf Salad

When your taste buds crave creamy, sweet, and crunchy, this salad fits the bill. This recipe is gluten-free.

2 Braeburn apples, peeled, cored, and chopped

1 Granny Smith apple, peeled, cored, and chopped

½ cup halved green grapes

½ cup chopped celery

½ cup raisins

½ cup chopped walnuts

½ cup Fresh-Made Mayonnaise (recipe earlier in this chapter)

¼ cup fat-free plain yogurt

2 TB. agave nectar

2 tsp. fresh lemon juice

⅛ tsp. fine sea salt

Yield: 10 servings
Prep time: 5 minutes
Chill time: 1 hour
Serving size: ½ cup
Each serving has:
224 calories
14 g fat
2 g saturated fat
23 g carbohydrates
2 g fiber
2 g protein
64 mg sodium

1. In a medium bowl, combine apples, grapes, celery, raisins, and walnuts.

2. In a small bowl, combine Fresh-Made Mayonnaise, yogurt, agave nectar, lemon juice, and sea salt. Stir to blend well. Pour over apple mixture, and stir to coat evenly.

3. Cover and chill for at least 1 hour before serving. Stir again before serving. Use within 5 days.

 For Good Measure

Commercially prepared mayonnaises are made with starches, sugars, and other additives. With a little practice, making mayonnaise at home is easy. Plus, you know exactly what ingredients are in it.

Summer Garden Coleslaw

The robust flavor of cabbage is blended with the sweet taste of green bell peppers and carrots in a lightly sweetened, creamy sauce. This recipe is gluten-free.

Yield: 6 servings
Prep time: 5 minutes
Chill time: 30 minutes
Serving size: ½ cup
Each serving has:
141 calories
11 g fat
2 g saturated fat
9 g carbohydrates
1 g fiber
1 g protein
35 mg sodium

3 cups shredded green cabbage

½ cup shredded green bell pepper

½ cup finely shredded carrots

⅓ cup Fresh-Made Mayonnaise (recipe earlier in this chapter)

2 TB. honey

⅛ tsp. ground mustard

⅛ tsp. garlic powder

⅛ tsp. onion powder

1. In a large bowl, combine cabbage, green bell pepper, and carrots.

2. In a small bowl, combine Fresh-Made Mayonnaise, honey, ground mustard, garlic powder, and onion powder. Stir until blended. Pour over cabbage mixture, and stir until evenly coated.

3. Cover and chill for at least 30 minutes before serving. Stir again to coat evenly before serving.

 Starch Guard

Choose a large bowl for mixing coleslaw. Even though this recipe makes 3 cups, the volume is greater when mixing; the cabbage wilts during chilling.

French-Flair Macaroni Salad

Quinoa elbow macaroni and crisp-tender steamed veggies are coated in a creamy sauce with a touch of Dijon and Gruyère cheese. This recipe is gluten-free.

1 (8-oz.) pkg. quinoa elbow pasta

1 cup 1-inch-cut fresh green beans

½ cup frozen peas

½ cup thinly sliced on the diagonal carrots

½ cup finely shredded Gruyère cheese

½ cup Fresh-Made Mayonnaise (recipe earlier in this chapter)

1 TB. Dijon mustard

1 TB. honey

Yield: 12 servings
Prep time: 15 minutes
Cook time: 9 minutes
Chill time: 1 hour
Serving size: ½ cup
Each serving has:
183 calories
10 g fat
2 g saturated fat
19 g carbohydrates
2 g fiber
4 g protein
79 mg sodium

1. Prepare quinoa pasta according to the package directions. Drain and rinse with cold water until cool.

2. Meanwhile, place green beans in a steamer basket over 1 inch of water. Cover and bring to a boil over high heat. Reduce heat to medium, and steam for 3 minutes. Carefully add peas and carrots to the steamer basket, cover, and steam for 2 minutes or until vegetables are crisp-tender. Remove from heat and cool.

3. In a large bowl, combine quinoa pasta, vegetables, and cheese.

4. In a small bowl, combine Fresh-Made Mayonnaise, Dijon mustard, and honey. Stir to blend well. Pour over quinoa pasta mixture, and stir until evenly coated.

5. Cover and chill for at least 1 hour before serving. Stir again before serving.

Variation: If you prefer very creamy macaroni salad, double the dressing, using 1 cup Fresh-Made Mayonnaise, 2 tablespoons Dijon mustard, and 2 tablespoons honey.

No-Flour Power

Cutting carrots on the diagonal provides more surface area for quicker cooking and offers a pretty presentation. To slice a carrot on the diagonal, hold the knife at a 45-degree angle to the carrot.

Tunisian Pasta Salad

The addition of cumin adds a new depth to the lemony Italian dressing that coats the al dente pasta, fresh veggies, and beans. This recipe is gluten-free.

Yield: 24 servings
Prep time: 5 minutes
Cook time: 10 minutes
Chill time: 8 hours
Serving size: ½ cup
Each serving has:
191 calories
12 g fat
2 g saturated fat
18 g carbohydrates
1 g fiber
2 g protein
25 mg sodium

1 (16-oz.) pkg. brown rice pasta springs

1 cup cooked garbanzo beans

1 cup diced tomatoes

½ cup diced green bell peppers

½ cup diced red bell peppers

¼ cup diced red onions

1 tsp. ground cumin

1¾ cups (1 recipe) Herb-Flecked Italian Dressing (recipe earlier in this chapter)

1. Prepare brown rice pasta according to the package directions, omitting any suggested salt and/or oil. Drain and rinse with cold water until cool.

2. In a 13×9×2 dish with a lid, combine garbanzo beans, tomatoes, green bell peppers, red bell peppers, and red onions. Add brown rice pasta, and stir to mix.

3. Whisk cumin into Herb-Flecked Italian Dressing until well blended. Pour over brown rice pasta mixture, and stir to coat evenly.

4. Cover and chill overnight. Stir well again before serving.

For Good Measure

Cooking dried beans is easy and saves on the sodium added during the processing of canned goods. Follow the package directions for the overnight or quick-soak methods.

Mexican Veggie Quinoa Salad

A light, refreshing salad full of Mexican-style flavors where the vegetables brighten in a lime-based dressing. This recipe is gluten-free.

2 cups cooked quinoa

1¾ cups cooked black beans or 1 (15.25-oz.) can black beans, rinsed and drained

1 cup frozen corn

1 cup finely chopped tomatoes

¼ cup sliced green onions

¼ cup finely chopped celery

1 TB. chopped fresh cilantro

1 large clove garlic, minced

¼ cup extra-virgin olive oil

¼ cup fresh lime juice

½ tsp. fine sea salt

⅛ tsp. freshly ground black pepper

⅛ tsp. hot pepper sauce

Yield: 10 servings
Prep time: 5 minutes
Chill time: 1 hour
Serving size: ½ cup
Each serving has:
241 calories
8 g fat
1 g saturated fat
35 g carbohydrates
5 g fiber
8 g protein
127 mg sodium

1. In a large bowl, combine quinoa, black beans, corn, tomatoes, green onions, celery, cilantro, and garlic. Stir to mix.

2. In a small bowl, combine extra-virgin olive oil, lime juice, sea salt, black pepper, and hot pepper sauce. Stir to blend. Pour over quinoa mixture, and stir to coat evenly.

3. Cover and chill for at least 1 hour before serving. Stir again before serving.

 For Good Measure _____

Quinoa (pronounced KEEN-WAH) is a small whole grain with a mild flavor. Quinoa can also be ground and used as a flourlike substitute.

Garlic-Pepper Croutons

Garlicky toasted cubes satisfy that craving for a spicy crunch in a green salad.

Yield: 8 servings
Prep time: 5 minutes
Cook time: 10 minutes
Serving size: 4 croutons
Each serving has:
34 calories
2 g fat
1 g saturated fat
4 g carbohydrates
1 g fiber
1 g protein
19 mg sodium

2 slices stale sprouted-grain bread

1 TB. unsalted butter, melted

2 medium cloves garlic, pressed

⅛ tsp. freshly ground black pepper

1. Preheat the oven to 350°F.

2. On a small nonstick baking pan, cut bread into 1-inch squares (16 pieces) without separating.

3. In a small bowl, stir together butter, garlic, and black pepper. Brush half of mixture over bread. Turn bread cubes, and brush remaining mixture on the other side.

4. Bake for 5 minutes. Turn bread cubes, and bake for 5 minutes more on the other side or until toasted. Let cool in the baking pan before serving.

For Good Measure

The recipes in this book call for unsalted butter to keep the sodium content as low as possible. Salted butter can be substituted, if you prefer.

Crispy Parmesan Snaps

Lacy, golden circles of baked Parmesan taste toasty and cheesy. This recipe is gluten-free.

¼ cup shredded Parmesan cheese

1. Preheat the oven to 350°F.

2. Line a large baking sheet with parchment paper. Spoon 1 teaspoon cheese onto the parchment paper, and using the back of the measuring spoon, flatten into a 2-inch lacy circle. Repeat for each snap, spacing 2 inches apart.

3. Bake for 4 to 5 minutes or until cheese is browned.

4. Cool on parchment paper for 1 to 2 minutes before peeling off to serve. Top green salads or toss into a bowl of soup.

Variation: For cheesier, less crisp snaps, reduce oven temperature to 300°F, and bake for 5 minutes or until lightly browned.

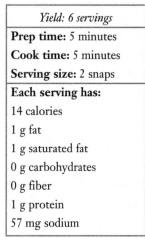

Yield: 6 servings
Prep time: 5 minutes
Cook time: 5 minutes
Serving size: 2 snaps
Each serving has:
14 calories
1 g fat
1 g saturated fat
0 g carbohydrates
0 g fiber
1 g protein
57 mg sodium

For Good Measure

Can wax paper be substituted for parchment paper in this recipe? No. Although both wax paper and parchment paper provide nonstick surfaces, only parchment paper can withstand the direct oven temperature.

11

Finger Food Favorites

In This Chapter

- Anytime finger-licking foods
- Always welcome no-utensils-necessary bites for gatherings
- Crowd-pleasing party snacks

Everyone loves noshes and nibbles. Tasty little tidbits find numerous takers at parties, family gatherings, get-togethers with friends, or just movie nights in front of the television. These fun foods, though, can traditionally be chock-full of flour and other unhealthful ingredients, so keep your fingers off!

Not to worry! You have better, more healthful options. The recipes here are flour-free and full of veggies, whole grains, and great taste.

Party Planning

When finger foods are party favorites, they're offered over a lengthy period of time. You need to do a little planning to keep the food safe.

Cold foods must be kept cold, and hot foods must be kept hot. Bowls or trays filled with crushed ice are good resting places for cold dishes that

Starch Guard

Foods held at room temperature for more than two hours must be thrown out. If your party is steaming hot—outdoors in temperatures above 90°F, that is—your food is only safe for one hour.

need to be held at or below 40°F. Hot foods can be served from slow cookers, chafing dishes, or warming trays to stay at or above 140°F.

With little fuss, you can simply serve finger foods in small amounts. Don't add fresh tidbits to the trays, though. Instead, exchange the serving dishes to be certain of the food's safety. Your guests will remember your smashing party, not their subsequent food-borne illness.

Oven-Fried Zucchini Fries

Tender strips of zucchini with a light cornmeal coating use up your garden bounty while satisfying your taste for fresh veggies. This recipe is gluten-free.

1 (7- to 8-inch) zucchini

3 TB. stone-ground yellow cornmeal

3 TB. stone-ground brown rice

4½ TB. water, or as needed

Yield: 6 servings
Prep time: 10 minutes
Cook time: 20 minutes
Serving size: about 8 fries
Each serving has:
39 calories
0 g fat
0 g saturated fat
8 g carbohydrates
1 g fiber
1 g protein
5 mg sodium

1. Preheat the oven to 400°F with the oven rack in the highest position.

2. Trim ends from zucchini and discard. Cut zucchini in half horizontally. Cut each half into ¼-inch *matchsticks*.

3. In a shallow dish, combine yellow cornmeal and stone-ground brown rice; stir. Add just enough water to moisten dry ingredients and make a thick paste.

4. Dredge zucchini matchsticks in cornmeal mixture to coat lightly. Arrange in a single layer on a large nonstick baking pan coated with cooking spray.

5. Bake for 10 minutes. Turn zucchini fries, and bake for 10 more minutes or until zucchini is tender and coating is crisp. Serve immediately.

Variation: Season the cornmeal with fine sea salt and freshly ground black pepper to taste.

 Words to Digest

Matchsticks refer to the shape of ingredients prepared by julienning. The food should be cut into long, thin strips.

Crispy Chicken Nuggets

Even the kids won't be able to resist these juicy white-meat morsels with their extra-crunchy coating.

Yield: 5 servings
Prep time: 10 minutes
Cook time: 15 minutes
Serving size: about 6 nuggets
Each serving has:
363 calories
12 g fat
6 g saturated fat
32 g carbohydrates
5 g fiber
33 g protein
235 mg sodium

1¼ lb. boneless, skinless chicken breasts, trimmed of fat

¼ cup unsalted butter, melted

2 cups sprouted-whole-grains cereal

1. Preheat the oven to 400°F.

2. Cut chicken breasts into 1½-inch pieces. Spread out into a shallow dish. Pour butter over top, and toss chicken to coat well.

3. Pour cereal into a large zipper-lock storage bag and close. Using a rolling pin or meat mallet, roll and/or crush cereal into crumbs. (Check the bag for holes before proceeding.)

4. Turn coated chicken pieces into the bag and shake to coat evenly. Arrange in a single layer on a large nonstick baking sheet coated with cooking spray. Bake for 15 minutes or until the internal temperature reads 170°F on a food thermometer.

No-Flour Power

Look for sprouted-whole-grains nugget cereal, such as Ezekiel 4:9, in your grocer's health-food section. See Appendix C for additional resources.

Baked Sweet Onion Rings

The sweet onion flavor comes through the light coating that provides a satisfying crunch.

1 large sweet onion	**½ tsp. fine sea salt**
1½ cups sprouted-grain breadcrumbs	**¼ tsp. freshly ground black pepper**
¼ cup chopped fresh parsley	**3 large egg whites**
¼ cup stone-ground brown rice	

Yield: 6 servings
Prep time: 12 minutes
Cook time: 20 minutes
Serving size: about 5 onion rings
Each serving has:
76 calories
0 g fat
0 g saturated fat
14 g carbohydrates
2 g fiber
4 g protein
240 mg sodium

1. Preheat the oven to 400°F. Move the oven rack to the highest position.

2. Cut sweet onion into ½-inch slices, and separate into rings. (Reserve smallest rings for another use.)

3. In a shallow dish, combine breadcrumbs and parsley; stir. In another shallow dish, combine stone-ground brown rice, sea salt, and black pepper; stir. In a third shallow dish, lightly beat egg whites.

4. Dredge onion rings in stone-ground brown rice mixture. Coat with egg whites. Dredge in breadcrumb mixture. Arrange in a single layer on a large nonstick baking sheet coated with cooking spray, placing smaller rings inside larger rings as needed.

5. Bake for 10 minutes. Turn and bake for 10 more minutes or until coating is crisp and onions are tender. Serve immediately.

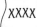 **No-Flour Power** _____

Egg yolks can be reserved to make Fresh-Made Mayonnaise (recipe in Chapter 10). To hold egg yolks, store them covered with a little water to mimic the whites in a tightly covered container. Refrigerate and use within 2 days, carefully removing the whole yolk with a spoon to use.

Ball-Park Mustard Deviled Eggs

Few ingredients make for easy preparation and a simple, uncomplicated, creamy deviled filling for hard-cooked eggs. This recipe is gluten-free.

Yield: 12 servings
Prep time: 20 minutes
Cook time: 30 minutes
Chill time: 30 minutes
Serving size: 1 egg half
Each serving has:
55 calories
5 g fat
1 g saturated fat
0 g carbohydrates
0 g fiber
3 g protein
50 mg sodium

6 large eggs

2 TB. Fresh-Made Mayonnaise (see Chapter 10)

1 TB. prepared yellow mustard

Ground paprika to taste

1. Fill a medium saucepan ¾ full with cold water. Carefully add eggs. Bring to a boil over high heat. Turn off heat. Cover and let stand for 20 minutes.

2. Remove eggs from hot water, and immediately rinse under cold, running water until cooled. Peel eggs.

3. Cut eggs in half lengthwise. Remove yolks to a medium bowl, and set aside whites.

4. Using the tines of a fork, break up yolks until fine crumbs form. Add Fresh-Made Mayonnaise and yellow mustard, and stir to blend.

5. Spoon or pipe yolk mixture into hollows of egg whites. Sprinkle paprika over tops. Chill for at least 30 minutes or until serving time. Refrigerate any leftovers, and use within 5 days.

 For Good Measure

Deviled eggs are a good use for the aging eggs in your fridge. Eggs can be used 3 to 5 weeks after the stamped sell-by date. Fresh eggs, though, aren't best for hard-cooking as they'll be nearly impossible to peel.

Cheesy Jalapeño Nachos

Smooth and cheesy, this sauce packs as much heat as you choose—
the more pepper seeds you include, the hotter—for topping the
subtle veggie-flavored, flaxseed-studded tortilla chips.

1 cup fat-free milk

**2 TB. stone-ground brown
rice**

**1 cup shredded sharp cheddar
cheese**

**2 medium jalapeño peppers,
seeded (optional) and finely
diced**

**1 (12-oz.) pkg. veggie
flaxseed tortilla chips**

Yield: 12 servings
Prep time: 2 minutes
Cook time: 5 minutes
Serving size: 7 tortilla chips with 2 tablespoons sauce
Each serving has:
193 calories
10 g fat
3 g saturated fat
20 g carbohydrates
3 g fiber
6 g protein
129 mg sodium

1. Pour milk into a medium saucepan. Whisk in stone-ground
   brown rice until smooth.

2. Cook over medium heat for 4 minutes or just until milk
   mixture starts to bubble, continually scraping the whisk over
   the bottom of the saucepan to keep milk from scorching.
   Immediately whisk in cheese for 1 minute or until melted.

3. Turn off heat. Continue to whisk until sauce is smooth. Stir in
   diced jalapeño peppers.

4. To serve, arrange tortilla chips on a large serving platter and
   pour cheese sauce over top; serve immediately. Or allow guests
   to dip tortilla chips into cheese sauce as desired.

Variation: If sodium is not a concern, stir a pinch or two of fine
sea salt into the sauce with the cheese.

Starch Guard

Processed, pre-shredded cheeses are packaged with
starches for their anti-caking properties. Opt for blocks of
natural cheeses you can shred, cube, or slice as needed.

Baked Buffalo Hot Wings

These "naked" wings allow you to skip the traditional breading and frying while still enjoying the flavor of smooth and spicy buffalo sauce. This recipe is gluten-free if the chicken is gluten-free.

Yield: 6 servings
Prep time: 5 minutes
Cook time: 40 minutes
Serving size: about 6 wings
Each serving has:
376 calories
20 g fat
9 g saturated fat
0 g carbohydrates
0 g fiber
50 g protein
586 mg sodium

3 lb. skinless chicken wing portions

6 TB. unsalted butter

4 TB. hot pepper sauce, or to taste

1. Preheat the oven to 425°F.

2. Arrange chicken wings on a large nonstick baking pan coated with cooking spray. Bake for 40 minutes or until internal temperature reads 180°F on a food thermometer.

3. Meanwhile, stir together melted butter and hot pepper sauce until blended.

4. Immediately remove chicken wings to a very large bowl. Pour butter mixture over all, and toss to coat evenly. Serve hot.

Variation: Substitute skin-on chicken wing portions if you prefer, but keep in mind the additional fat and calories.

No-Flour Power

To read the wings' temperature accurately, place the probe of a food thermometer in a meaty portion of a chicken wing. Take care not to touch a bone or the baking pan.

Flat Bread Dough

Enjoy a chewy, medium-thick crust when baked. This recipe is gluten-free.

2 cups stone-ground brown rice

½ cup stone-ground yellow cornmeal

2 TB. xanthan gum

1½ tsp. fine sea salt

½ tsp. freshly ground black pepper

1 (¼-oz.) pkg. active dry yeast (about 2¼ tsp.)

¾ cup plus ½ cup warm water (105°F to 110°F)

2 TB. extra-virgin olive oil

Yield: 8 servings
Prep time: 1½ hours
Cook time: 30 minutes
Serving size: 2⅜×3⅜-inch square
Each serving has:
216 calories
5 g fat
1 g saturated fat
39 g carbohydrates
5 g fiber
4 g protein
432 mg sodium

1. In a medium bowl, combine stone-ground brown rice, yellow cornmeal, xanthan gum, sea salt, and black pepper. Stir, and make a well in the center.

2. Dissolve yeast in ¾ cup warm water until it bubbles (about 5 minutes). Pour into well of dry ingredients.

3. Pull dry ingredients into wet ingredients to moisten as much as possible. Drizzle in ½ cup warm water, and stir to moisten all dry ingredients. Add extra-virgin olive oil, and stir to blend well, pulling into a ball and cleaning the side of the bowl.

4. Turn out dough onto a work surface dusted with stone-ground brown rice. Turn dough over, working into a ball with your hands.

5. Transfer dough to a large bowl coated with cooking spray, turning over to coat dough. Cover with a clean dish towel, and let rise in a warm place for 1 hour or until dough has risen a bit and feels spongy. (Let rise in the oven with the light on if an 85°F, draft-free area is unavailable.)

6. Turn out dough onto a work surface dusted with stone-ground brown rice. Using dusted hands, flatten dough, pushing edges back in as they separate. Turn dough over and flatten again.

7. Transfer dough to a large cookie sheet (without a rim) coated with cooking spray. Roll dough into a 13½×9½-inch rectangle, pushing edges in to form a small rim around edges. Let dough rest while the oven preheats.

Starch Guard

Use a thermometer to test the temperature of the warm water when proofing dry yeast. Too hot, and the heat will kill the live yeast.

8. Preheat the oven to 375°F. Bake dough for 30 minutes or until crust is golden brown. Transfer to a wire rack to cool. Top as you would a pizza dough. (Try the following recipe for Flat Bread Taco Pizza, or use the recipe as a guideline for topping and baking as you prefer.)

Flat Bread Taco Pizza

A chewy crust holds warm taco filling favorites for a tasty tidbit.
This recipe is gluten-free.

1 prepared Flat Bread Dough (recipe earlier in this chapter)

1 cup fat-free refried beans

½ cup shredded sharp cheddar cheese

½ cup shredded Colby-Monterey Jack cheese

½ cup *diced*, seeded tomatoes (about 1 medium)

⅓ cup sliced black olives (about 8 extra-large)

¼ cup diced red onions

1 cup shredded romaine lettuce

Yield: 16 servings
Prep time: 8 minutes
Cook time: 10 minutes
Serving size: 2 squares
Each serving has:
158 calories
6 g fat
2 g saturated fat
22 g carbohydrates
3 g fiber
5 g protein
352 mg sodium

1. Preheat the oven to 350°F.

2. Place prepared Flat Bread Dough on a medium nonstick baking sheet. Spread refried beans evenly over crust up to the raised edge. Sprinkle on cheddar cheese, Colby-Monterey Jack cheese, tomatoes, black olives, and red onions.

3. Bake for 7 minutes. Sprinkle lettuce evenly over all. Bake for 3 minutes or until cheese is bubbly and toppings are heated through.

4. Let pizza stand for 5 minutes before cutting. Using a pizza cutter, cut pizza into about 2⅜×1⅞-inch squares (32 squares) to serve.

Variation: Cut pizza into 16 squares to serve.

Words to Digest

Diced is a way of cutting ingredients into small cubes that are about ¼-inch square.

Garbanzo and Fava Cracker Crisps

Lightly bean-flavored, these bite-size crackers serve up garlic-salted tops and a crisp crunch. This recipe is gluten-free.

Yield: 15 servings
Prep time: 15 minutes
Cook time: 20 to 24 minutes
Serving size: about 12 crackers
Each serving has:
90 calories
3 g fat
1 g saturated fat
11 g carbohydrates
3 g fiber
4 g protein
189 mg sodium

1½ cups ground garbanzo and fava beans	1 large egg, at room temperature
1 cup puréed cooked garbanzo beans	2 TB. extra-virgin olive oil
3 TB. grated fresh Parmesan cheese	2 TB. fresh lemon juice
	½ tsp. garlic powder
1 tsp. baking soda	½ tsp. fine sea salt

1. Preheat the oven to 425°F.

2. In a large bowl, combine 1 cup ground garbanzo and fava beans, puréed garbanzo beans, Parmesan cheese, and baking soda. Stir to mix.

3. In a small bowl, whisk egg until lemon-colored. Add extra-virgin olive oil and lemon juice, and stir to blend. Pour into bean mixture, and stir until dry ingredients are moistened. Work in ¼ cup ground garbanzo and fava beans until moistened. Divide dough in half.

4. Dust a work surface with 2 tablespoons ground garbanzo and fava beans. Coat half of dough with ground beans to keep surface dry while working dough into a rectangle with dusted hands, flipping dough and flattening into a rectangle. Dust the work surface with additional ground beans as needed to keep dough from sticking. Dust a rolling pin, and roll dough ⅛-inch thick (about a 13×7-inch rectangle).

5. Carefully transfer to a medium or large nonstick baking pan coated with cooking spray. With a knife, deeply score dough into 1-inch squares. Sprinkle ¼ teaspoon garlic powder and ¼ teaspoon sea salt over top. Bake for 10 to 12 minutes or until browned well, dry, and crisp. Let cool on the baking pan.

6. Meanwhile, roll out remaining dough on the work surface dusted with remaining 2 tablespoons ground beans. Repeat the rolling out, transferring, scoring, seasoning, and baking directions given.

7. When cooled, break baked dough into crackers along score lines. Store in an airtight container.

No-Flour Power

To achieve the 1 cup puréed, cooked garbanzo beans called for in this recipe, place 1 cup whole cooked garbanzo beans in a blender. Cover and purée on high until beans are very finely chopped. (They'll be dry, not a wet purée.)

Party Munchies Mix

This snack mix satisfies everyone's craving for a crunchy and spicy nibble. This recipe is gluten-free.

1½ cups cooked garbanzo beans

2 TB. extra-virgin olive oil

½ tsp. garlic powder

½ tsp. onion powder

¼ tsp. cayenne pepper

⅛ tsp. fine sea salt

½ cup sea-salted cocktail peanuts

½ cup broken to bite-size wheat-free, gluten-free herb crackers (about 13)

Yield: *9 servings*
Prep time: 5 minutes
Cook time: 30 minutes
Serving size: ¼ cup
Each serving has:
188 calories
12 g fat
2 g saturated fat
13 g carbohydrates
4 g fiber
7 g protein
117 mg sodium

1. Preheat the oven to 450°F.

2. In a medium bowl, combine garbanzo beans, extra-virgin olive oil, garlic powder, onion powder, cayenne pepper, and sea salt. Stir to coat evenly.

3. Spread coated garbanzo beans into a single layer on a small nonstick baking pan, pouring any olive oil that clings to the bowl over beans. Bake for 30 minutes or until crisped, stirring halfway through baking time. Cool slightly.

4. In a medium serving bowl, combine garbanzo beans, cocktail peanuts, and herb crackers. Serve immediately.

XXXX No-Flour Power

Check your grocer's special dietary needs aisle for wheat-free, gluten-free crackers, such as the Mary's Gone Crackers line. Or turn to Appendix C for a list of resources.

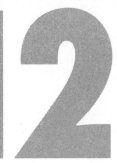

Appealing Appetizers

In This Chapter

- ◆ Delectable dinner party pick-ups and plated starters
- ◆ Flavorful flourless substitutes
- ◆ Delicious dips for flour-free scoops

Some of us don't need any help getting ready to eat, but we're fond of appetizers just the same. A delicious start to a meal can offer variety in a small package.

You don't have to limit yourself to the veggie tray, though. Eliminating flour or substituting for it keeps your appetizers healthful and your blood glucose levels in check. Plus, cultivating a new take on how foods are served will open a plethora of possibilities for your next dinner party.

Sizing Up a Serving

Look at any nutrition data box or the nutrition analysis next to each recipe in this cookbook and you'll find valuable information for your health. If you ignore the serving size listed, though, you may as well not waste your time. All the information is based on the given serving size.

Appetizers are aptly named, as they are intended to whet your appetite. Unless you're at a *tapas* bar, you'll probably eat a full meal following. Just trying a bit of each appetizer likely fulfills the serving size, but eating more than one serving is so easy to do. Follow the provided nutrition information for an appetizer-size portion. Of course, you can indulge in more than one serving if you like, even make a main meal of your favorites, but please do so consciously.

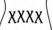

No-Flour Power

Comparing nutrition labels can't always be done at a glance. When evaluating similar products against one another, don't assume the information is based on the same serving size. You'll need to calculate the difference, if necessary, and it might surprise you. A 1 cup serving size with 200 calories is lower in overall calories than a 6-ounce serving with 175 calories.

Buffalo-Style Stuffed Mushroom Caps

The fiery feel of wing sauce mingled with its classic accompaniments—blue cheese and celery—livens up meaty mushroom bites. This recipe is gluten-free.

Yield: 10 servings
Prep time: 10 minutes
Cook time: 22 minutes
Serving size: 3 mushroom caps

1 TB. unsalted butter

¼ cup finely diced celery

3 oz. Neufchâtel cheese or reduced-fat cream cheese

1 cup crumbled blue cheese

2 TB. hot pepper sauce or to taste

30 medium white button mushrooms, stems removed

Each serving has:
99 calories
7 g fat
4 g saturated fat
4 g carbohydrates
0 g fiber
6 g protein
318 mg sodium

1. Preheat the oven to 350°F.

2. In a small skillet, melt butter over medium heat. Stir in celery. Cook, stirring often, for 5 minutes or until softened. Remove from heat, and cool for 3 minutes.

3. In a medium bowl, combine Neufchâtel cheese, blue cheese, and hot pepper sauce. Stir to blend. Add celery mixture, and stir to mix.

4. Spoon cheese mixture into hollows of mushroom caps. Arrange stuffed mushrooms on a large nonstick baking sheet. Bake for 15 minutes or until mushrooms are softened and release liquid. Serve hot.

No-Flour Power

Clean mushrooms with a mushroom brush or a soft-bristled toothbrush. If mushrooms need washing to remove dirt, you can clean them quickly under gently running water. Mushrooms absorb water, so they shouldn't be soaked or they will become water-logged.

Roasted Cheddar and Cream Cheese Poppers

These "naked" poppers allow the crisp, fresh pepper taste to mingle with the toasted, gooey, double-cheesy filling. This recipe is gluten-free.

Yield: 6 servings
Prep time: 15 minutes
Cook time: 5 minutes
Serving size: 2 poppers
Each serving has:
166 calories
14 g fat
9 g saturated fat
2 g carbohydrates
0 g fiber
9 g protein
247 mg sodium

6 medium fresh jalapeño peppers

1¼ cups shredded cheddar cheese

4 oz. Neufchâtel cheese or reduced-fat cream cheese

¼ cup chopped fresh cilantro

1. Preheat the oven to 425°F.

2. Halve each jalapeño pepper lengthwise, leaving stem intact for presentation, if desired. Cut out seeds and white membranes. (Clean out jalapeño peppers very well for the mildest taste or retain some seeds and membranes for a fiery flavor.)

3. In a small bowl, stir together cheddar cheese, Neufchâtel cheese, and cilantro. Blend until evenly distributed.

4. Spoon cheese mixture by heaping tablespoonfuls into jalapeño pepper halves, pressing into depressions. Arrange on a baking sheet, and bake for 5 minutes or until cheese is bubbly and undersides of jalapeño peppers are starting to char.

Starch Guard

Use caution when preparing fresh hot peppers. The capsaicin can burn your skin and irritate your eyes and nose. Wash your hands immediately afterward. If you're very sensitive, you may want to wear latex gloves.

Belgian Endive Stuffed with Cucumber Salad

Cool and crisp, this simple salad is delivered in an edible container that offers guests a refreshing start to their meals, rather than heavy, starchy bread. This recipe is gluten-free.

2 cups finely diced cucumber (about 1 medium)

1 cup finely diced seeded tomato (about 1 large)

¼ cup minced red onion

¼ cup reduced-fat sour cream

1 tsp. fresh lemon juice

¼ tsp. celery seeds

¼ tsp. fine sea salt

¼ tsp. freshly ground black pepper

20 whole Belgian endive leaves

Yield: 10 servings		
Prep time: 10 minutes		
Chill time: 1 hour		
Serving size: 2 stuffed leaves		
Each serving has:		
19 calories		
1 g fat		
1 g saturated fat		
3 g carbohydrates		
1 g fiber		
0 g protein		
59 mg sodium		

1. In a medium bowl, combine cucumber, tomato, red onion, sour cream, lemon juice, celery seeds, sea salt, and black pepper. Stir to coat evenly. Cover and chill for at least 1 hour before serving.

2. Using a slotted spoon, fill each endive leaf with 2 tablespoons cucumber mixture. Serve immediately.

Variation: Peel and seed the cucumber, if you prefer, or substitute the same amount of seedless English cucumber.

 Starch Guard

Anytime you're eating the peel of produce, organic or otherwise, wash it well. Using a commercial fruit and vegetable wash is easy and effective.

Broiled Tomatoes with Herb Crumb Topping

These fresh-tasting tomatoes are delectable served warm and juicy with a perfectly seasoned, crunchy topping.

Yield: 6 servings
Prep time: 3 minutes
Cook time: 4 minutes
Serving size: 1 tomato half
Each serving has:
38 calories
1 g fat
0 g saturated fat
6 g carbohydrates
1 g fiber
2 g protein
90 mg sodium

3 medium ripe tomatoes

½ cup sprouted-grain bread-crumbs

2 TB. shredded Parmesan cheese

1 TB. chopped fresh basil

1 TB. chopped fresh oregano

⅛ tsp. fine sea salt

⅛ tsp. freshly ground black pepper

1. Preheat the broiler on high.

2. Core tomatoes and cut in half horizontally. Arrange cut side up on a nonstick baking pan coated with cooking spray. (Trim bottoms of tomatoes, if needed, to allow tomato halves to sit level.)

3. Combine sprouted-grain breadcrumbs, Parmesan cheese, basil, oregano, sea salt, and black pepper in a small bowl. Stir to mix.

4. Broil tomato halves 4 inches from heat for 1 to 2 minutes or until softened slightly. Top each tomato half with 2 tablespoons breadcrumb mixture, spreading to the edge of tomato halves. Broil for an additional 1 to 2 minutes or until topping is golden brown, watching closely to keep from burning. Serve immediately.

No-Flour Power _____

To make sprouted-grain breadcrumbs, simply tear a slice of sprouted-grain, flourless bread into small pieces, and place them in a blender. Cover and blend on high speed for 5 to 10 seconds or until small crumbs form. A slice of sprouted-grain bread yields about ¾ cup of crumbs.

Fried Green Tomatoes

This crisp cornmeal coating encloses the tart taste of the underripe fruit for an end-of-harvest treat. This recipe is gluten-free.

4 large green tomatoes	**½ tsp. fine sea salt**
1½ cups stone-ground yellow cornmeal	**½ tsp. freshly ground black pepper**
½ cup ground garbanzo and fava beans	**2 large eggs, at room temperature**

1. Core tomatoes. Trim both ends to create a fairly flat cooking surface. Slice tomatoes about ⅜-inch thick.

2. In a shallow dish, combine yellow cornmeal, ground garbanzo and fava beans, sea salt, and black pepper. Stir to mix thoroughly.

3. In another shallow dish, whisk eggs until lemon-colored.

4. Heat a large nonstick skillet over medium heat. When the skillet is hot, coat with cooking spray.

5. Dip a tomato slice in egg, allowing excess to drip off. *Dredge* in cornmeal mixture to coat completely, shaking off excess. Fry coated tomato slices in batches, not crowding the skillet.

6. Cook on the first side for 3 to 4 minutes or until golden on the bottom. Quickly coat each tomato slice with cooking spray, and turn to cook the other side. Cook for 2 to 3 minutes or until underside is browned. Again, quickly coat each tomato slice with cooking spray. Turn to cook the first side for 1 minute more or until browned. Serve hot.

Yield: 8 servings
Prep time: 10 minutes
Cook time: 6 to 8 minutes per batch
Serving size: ½ tomato (about 4 slices)
Each serving has:
178 calories
5 g fat
1 g saturated fat
28 g carbohydrates
4 g fiber
6 g protein
179 mg sodium

Words to Digest

Dredge refers to covering a piece of food with a dry substance, such as a flour substitute or cornmeal.

Turkey-and-Swiss-Topped Cucumber Rounds

An icy cucumber slice serves as a crisp bed for the Swiss cheese and fresh turkey slices enlivened by a touch of Dijonnaise sauce.

Yield: 12 servings
Prep time: 6 minutes
Cook time: 12 to 14 minutes
Serving size: 2 rounds
Each serving has:
50 calories
3 g fat
1 g saturated fat
1 g carbohydrates
0 g fiber
6 g protein
317 mg sodium

1 (6.5-oz.) boneless, skinless turkey breast fillet

¼ tsp. fine sea salt

¼ tsp. freshly ground black pepper

1 medium cucumber, sliced ¼-inch thick

4 thin slices reduced-fat Swiss cheese (about 3×3½-inches)

1 TB. Fresh-Made Mayonnaise (see Chapter 10)

1 TB. Dijon mustard

1. Heat a medium skillet over medium heat. When hot, coat skillet with cooking spray.

2. Season both sides of turkey breast with sea salt and black pepper. Cook for 6 to 7 minutes on each side, turning once, or until the internal temperature reads 170°F on a food thermometer. Remove from the skillet and let stand.

3. Arrange cucumber slices on a large tray. Cut each cheese slice into 6 squares. Top each cucumber slice with a piece of cheese.

4. In a small bowl, combine Fresh-Made Mayonnaise and Dijon mustard. Stir until blended. Dollop ¼ teaspoon on each cheese slice.

5. Thinly slice turkey breast into strips. Layer turkey strips on top of Fresh-Made Mayonnaise mixture at a diagonal to cheese slices.

6. Serve immediately, or chill until serving time. Refrigerate any leftovers, and use within 5 days.

Starch Guard

Scan the Dijon mustard labels before making your purchase. Many brands add sugars and starches.

Cocktail Turkey BBQ Meatballs

Baked turkey meatballs with a hint of rosemary are coated in a spiced red tomato sauce sweetened with honey. This recipe is gluten-free.

1.2 lb. ground turkey breast

2 large eggs at room temperature, beaten

¼ cup minced sweet onion

1 tsp. garlic powder

1 tsp. fine sea salt

1 tsp. freshly ground black pepper

½ tsp. dried crushed rosemary

1⅛ cups Honey Barbecue Sauce (recipe later in this chapter)

Yield: 19 servings
Prep time: 10 minutes
Cook time: 20 minutes
Serving size: 2 meatballs
Each serving has:
61 calories
1 g fat
0 g saturated fat
6 g carbohydrates
0 g fiber
7 g protein
637 mg sodium

1. Preheat the oven to 400°F.

2. In a large bowl, combine turkey breast, eggs, sweet onion, garlic powder, sea salt, black pepper, and rosemary. Stir or use your hands to mix. Roll into 1-inch balls.

3. Arrange meatballs on a large nonstick baking pan coated with cooking spray. Bake for 20 minutes or until the internal temperature reads 170°F on a food thermometer.

4. Meanwhile, pour Honey Barbecue Sauce into a small slow cooker. Cover and heat on low.

5. Add meatballs to slow cooker when done, and stir gently to coat. Serve from slow cooker set on low to keep warm with toothpicks nearby, or spoon onto a serving platter and place a toothpick in each meatball.

 For Good Measure

Meatball recipes often call for breadcrumbs, cracker crumbs, or soup mixes so you can't assume that every meatball is flour-free.

Honey Barbecue Sauce

This tomato-based barbecue sauce is sweet and spicy. This recipe is gluten-free.

Yield: 9 servings
Prep time: 2 minutes
Serving size: 2 table-spoons
Each serving has:
45 calories
0 g fat
0 g saturated fat
11 g carbohydrates
1 g fiber
0 g protein
216 mg sodium

6 TB. tomato paste
¼ cup water
¼ cup cider vinegar
¼ cup honey
1 tsp. paprika

½ tsp. garlic powder
½ tsp. onion powder
½ tsp. fine sea salt
¼ tsp. hot pepper sauce

1. In a medium bowl, combine tomato paste, water, cider vinegar, honey, paprika, garlic powder, onion powder, sea salt, and hot pepper sauce. Stir until well blended.

2. To use as a dipping sauce, heat through. Or use as a baste—but keep in mind its honey content, and only baste foods during the last 5 to 10 minutes of cooking time.

Starch Guard

The honey adds natural sugars to this barbecue sauce, which will cause burning if cooked for too long at high temperatures.

Fresh-Taste Tomato Salsa

Balanced between chunky and saucy, this salsa's cilantro and lime juice highlight its south-of-the-border flair. This recipe is gluten-free.

4 medium tomatoes

1 cup finely chopped tomatoes

½ cup diced red onion

½ cup chopped fresh cilantro

1 medium jalapeño pepper, seeded (optional) and minced

3 TB. fresh lime juice

1 tsp. fine sea salt

Yield: 15 servings
Prep time: 5 minutes
Chill time: 1 hour
Serving size: ¼ cup
Each serving has:
16 calories
0 g fat
0 g saturated fat
3 g carbohydrates
1 g fiber
1 g protein
154 mg sodium

1. Core 4 medium tomatoes. Cut in half horizontally, and seed by squeezing each half over a bowl or the sink until seeds are released; discard seeds.

2. Place tomato halves in a blender. Cover and purée on high for 20 seconds or until desired consistency is reached.

3. In a medium bowl, combine puréed tomatoes, chopped tomatoes, red onion, cilantro, jalapeño pepper, lime juice, and sea salt. Stir until blended.

4. Cover and chill for at least 1 hour before serving. Stir again before serving.

Variation: For added heat, retain the seeds in the jalapeño pepper and add more jalapeño peppers as desired.

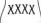 **No-Flour Power** _____

To extract the most juice from a lime (or other citrus fruit), roll the lime on the counter under the heel of your hand before cutting.

Red Bell Pepper Hummus

The fresh sweetness of a red bell pepper provides a pleasant undertone for the spicy bean paste. This recipe is gluten-free.

Yield: 14 servings
Prep time: 10 minutes
Serving size: 2 table-spoons
Each serving has:
39 calories
1 g fat
0 g saturated fat
7 g carbohydrates
2 g fiber
2 g protein
41 mg sodium

1 medium red bell pepper, seeded and chopped

1¾ cups cooked garbanzo beans

3 medium cloves garlic

½ tsp. ground cumin

¼ tsp. fine sea salt

3 TB. water

2 TB. fresh lemon juice

1. Combine red bell pepper, garbanzo beans, garlic cloves, cumin, sea salt, water, and lemon juice in a blender. Cover and blend on high speed for 5 minutes or until mixture is a thick paste and ingredients are blended. Stop to scrape down sides and redistribute ingredients frequently.

2. Serve immediately, or chill until serving time. Refrigerate any leftovers. Serve with veggie dippers—carrot sticks, cucumber slices, fresh snow peas—or with Garbanzo and Fava Cracker Crisps (see Chapter 11), or enjoy as a sandwich spread.

No-Flour Power

You don't have to resort to bottled lemon juice. Always keep fresh lemon juice on hand—in your freezer. Wash fresh lemons, cut into wedges, and toss into a freezer storage bag or airtight container. Thaw the wedges as needed—and, yes, you can pop them in the microwave for a few seconds to take the chill off.

Quick and Cheesy Quesadillas

Hearty corn tortillas enclose the taste of melted cheese and fresh salsa. This recipe is gluten-free.

6 prepared Fold-Over Corn Tortillas (see Chapter 8)

¾ cup shredded Colby-Monterey Jack cheese

6 TB. Fresh-Taste Tomato Salsa (recipe earlier in this chapter)

Yield: 6 servings
Prep time: 2 minutes
Cook time: 12 minutes
Serving size: 2 quarters
Each serving has:
193 calories
6 g fat
3 g saturated fat
27 g carbohydrates
3 g fiber
7 g protein
330 mg sodium

1. Heat a large nonstick skillet over medium heat. When the skillet is hot, coat with cooking spray.

2. Prepare each quesadilla by layering 1 Fold-Over Corn Tortilla, ¼ cup cheese, 2 tablespoons salsa, and 1 Fold-Over Corn Tortilla.

3. Cook quesadillas, 1 at a time, for 2 minutes or until cheese starts to melt. Turn and cook for 2 more minutes or until underside is browned and cheese is bubbly.

4. Remove from skillet to cool slightly. Cut into quarters to serve. Serve with sour cream and/or guacamole, if desired.

 No-Flour Power

A pizza cutter rolls right through these thicker quesadillas, making serving easy.

Part 4

Mealtime Makeovers

Now that you've thrown out all your flour sacks, maybe the most dreaded question is, "What's for dinner?" But the answer is easy. Mouthwatering meals!

All your favorites can still be enjoyed—beef, pork, fish and seafood, pasta, meatless main dishes, vegetables, sauces and gravies, and casseroles. With a variety of ingredients and a range of preparation times, you'll find recipes to please your pickiest eaters.

Meaty Entrées

In This Chapter

- ◆ Hearty beef and pork dishes to satisfy any appetite
- ◆ Tasty chicken and turkey meals for poultry lovers
- ◆ Spicy seasoning and marinade to flavor your favorites

Preparing meats, poultry, and fish at home requires steps to ensure safety. From supermarket to refrigerator to table, safe food handling remains vital. A little know-how makes it easy for you to stay safe from food-borne illnesses—and well fed.

For Safe Keeping

Safe handling starts in the supermarket. Most stores supply plastic bags for holding your raw meat purchases. For the utmost safety, slip your hand into the plastic bag, turning it inside out. Then, using the covered hand, pick up your preferred package and pull the bag right side out around it. Any raw meat juices should be caught, keeping your other purchases safe in the shopping cart and on the trip home.

When you get home—where you should go immediately following grocery shopping—store your raw meats, poultry, and fish on the lowest refrigerator shelf. Not only should this be the coldest part of your refrigerator, but any leaks will be contained from contaminating foods on lower shelves. Beef and pork cuts can be stored for 3 to 4 days. Poultry and ground meats should be used in 2 days. Fresh fish and seafood should be prepared in just a day or two. Freeze otherwise.

For Good Measure

Fish and seafood can be cooked to sight. Finfish should be opaque and flake easily with a fork. Shrimp will turn opaque and rosy pink.

Use a food thermometer to check for doneness when cooking, as the internal temperature is the only sure way to verify thorough cooking of meats and poultry. Suggested temperatures may appear on your food thermometer for easy reference, or use the chart here as a guide.

Recommended Cooking Temperatures

Ground Meats and Poultry	
Ground beef, pork, or veal	160°F
Ground chicken or turkey	165°F
Beef	
Medium rare	145°F
Medium	160°F
Well done	170°F
Pork	
Medium	160°F
Well done	170°F
Poultry	
Breasts or roasts	170°F
Whole chicken or turkey	180°F
Thighs, wings, or legs	180°F
Egg dishes	160°F
Stuffing	165°F
Leftovers	165°F

Chipotle Beef Fork-Style Fajitas

Thin slices of steak seasoned with the smoky flavor of chipotle chili pepper stuff a hearty corn tortilla along with green peppers, onions, tomatoes, and cheddar. This recipe is gluten-free.

¾ lb. thin-cut bottom round steak

½ tsp. chipotle chili pepper seasoning

½ large green bell pepper, cut into strips

½ medium yellow onion, sliced

2 medium cloves garlic, minced

¼ tsp. ground cumin

2 tsp. chopped fresh cilantro

1½ tsp. chopped fresh basil

½ cup diced tomatoes

4 Fold-Over Corn Tortillas (see Chapter 8)

½ cup shredded cheddar cheese

Yield: 4 servings
Prep time: 8 minutes
Cook time: 26 minutes
Serving size: 1 fajita
Each serving has:
331 calories
12 g fat
5 g saturated fat
31 g carbohydrates
4 g fiber
26 g protein
353 mg sodium

1. Preheat the oven to 350°F.

2. Cut steak into strips, and season with chipotle chili pepper.

3. Heat a large skillet over medium heat. When hot, add steak. Cook and stir for 4 minutes or until just browned on both sides. Drain.

4. Return the skillet to the heat. Stir in green bell pepper strips, onion slices, garlic, and cumin. Cook, stirring frequently, for 7 minutes or until vegetables are tender.

5. Turn off heat. Stir in cilantro, basil, and tomatoes. Divide mixture evenly among Fold-Over Corn Tortillas, spooning down centers. Sprinkle cheese over top.

6. Arrange stuffed tortillas in an 8×8×2 baking dish coated with cooking spray, setting upright as for tacos. Bake, uncovered, for 15 minutes or until cheese is melted and tortillas are crisped. Serve hot.

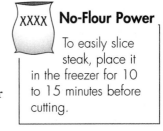

No-Flour Power

XXXX   To easily slice steak, place it in the freezer for 10 to 15 minutes before cutting.

Variation: Substitute an equal amount of another thin-sliced steak. Sprinkle cheese on after fajitas are baked if you prefer it freshly melted.

Tri-Color Peppers and Onions Smothered Steak

This tender broiled steak is accompanied by colorful bell peppers and onions with their sweet roasted flavor. This recipe is gluten-free.

Yield: 4 servings
Prep time: 35 minutes
Chill time: 8 hours
Cook time: 31 to 33 minutes
Serving size: 1 piece steak plus ¾ cup peppers and onions
Each serving has:
212 calories
7 g fat
2 g saturated fat
13 g carbohydrates
3 g fiber
26 g protein
78 mg sodium

1 lb. 1-inch-thick top sirloin steak, trimmed of fat

1 cup Vim and Vinegar Marinade (recipe later in this chapter)

1 large green bell pepper

1 medium red bell pepper

1 medium yellow bell pepper

1 large yellow onion

1 tsp. extra-virgin olive oil

1. Prick steak with the tines of a fork, and place steak in a zipper-lock bag. Pour Vim and Vinegar Marinade into the bag, and seal, pressing out air. Turn under the top of the bag to concentrate marinade over steak. Refrigerate for 8 hours or overnight, turning once if possible.

2. Preheat the broiler on high with the oven rack positioned 5 inches from the heating element.

3. Arrange whole green bell pepper, red bell pepper, and yellow bell pepper on a small nonstick baking sheet. Quarter onion, and arrange on the baking sheet. Brush extra-virgin olive oil over all onion surfaces. Broil for 15 minutes, turning bell peppers with tongs every 5 minutes to char all sides.

4. Transfer each bell pepper to a brown paper bag, and close bags loosely. When cool enough to handle (about 20 minutes), remove each pepper from each bag, 1 at a time. Cut open over a serving bowl to catch the juices. On a cutting board, core and seed each pepper and cut away white membranes. Peel off skin. Cut each pepper into strips. Add to the serving bowl with onions, separating into petals. Stir, and keep warm.

5. Adjust the oven rack to broil steak 6 inches from the heating element. Discard marinade, and place steak on a broiler pan coated with cooking spray. Cut deep vertical slits into edges of steak about every 2 inches to keep edges from curling up during cooking. Broil for 10 minutes or until top is browned.

Turn and broil for 6 to 8 minutes or until the temperature on a food thermometer reads 160°F for medium. Let steak stand for 5 minutes before cutting.

6. To serve, cut steak into 4 equal pieces. Top each piece with ¾ cup peppers and onions mixture.

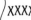

No-Flour Power

Read your broiler's instruction manual for recommendations. Electric stoves should have the oven door positioned ajar at the first stop-point when the broiler is in use to prevent the oven from overheating.

Vim and Vinegar Marinade

This red wine vinegar-based marinade forgoes the oil and adds a bit of heat and herbs. This recipe is gluten-free.

Yield: 1 cup
Prep time: 2 minutes
Each recipe has:
11 calories
0 g fat
0 g saturated fat
2 g carbohydrates
0 g fiber
0 g protein
12 mg sodium

⅔ cup water

⅓ cup red wine vinegar

1 medium clove garlic, thinly sliced

½ tsp. onion powder

¼ tsp. cayenne pepper

¼ tsp. ground dried thyme

1. In a measuring cup or a small bowl, combine water, red wine vinegar, garlic, onion powder, cayenne pepper, and thyme. Stir to mix.

2. To use, pour over meats or vegetables. Marinate in the refrigerator.

Starch Guard

Marinate in the refrigerator to prevent harmful bacterial growth. Discard all marinade that has been in contact with raw meats.

Fiesta Chicken Taco Salad

Mildly spicy chicken strips are bedded by lettuce, cheddar, and tortilla chips for a Tex-Mex favorite.

1 lb. boneless, skinless chicken breasts, trimmed of fat

4 tsp. Taco Seasoning Blend (recipe later in this chapter)

½ cup water

4 cups torn leaf lettuce

1 cup chopped tomatoes

1 cup shredded cheddar cheese

¼ cup sliced black olives

¼ cup diced red onions

36 unsalted yellow corn baked tortilla chips

Yield: 4 servings
Prep time: 5 minutes
Cook time: 13 to 14 minutes
Serving size: 1 salad
Each serving has:
349 calories
15 g fat
8 g saturated fat
17 g carbohydrates
3 g fiber
37 g protein
607 mg sodium

1. Heat a large skillet over medium heat. When hot, coat with cooking spray.

2. Meanwhile, cut chicken breasts into ¾-inch strips. Add chicken to the skillet. Cook for 3 to 4 minutes, turning to brown all sides. Sprinkle Taco Seasoning Blend over chicken, and pour water over top. Cook, stirring occasionally, for 10 minutes or until skillet is nearly dry. Remove from the heat and stir to coat chicken evenly.

3. Arrange lettuce, tomatoes, cheese, black olives, red onions, and tortilla chips on 4 plates, dividing evenly. Top with chicken strips, dividing evenly. Serve with reduced-fat sour cream, guacamole, Fresh-Taste Tomato Salsa (see Chapter 12), and/or Really Ranch Dressing (see Chapter 10), as desired.

Starch Guard

Keep a separate cutting board available for cutting raw meat, poultry, and fish. Plus, remember to wash everything that comes in contact with raw meats—the cutting board, utensils, your hands—with warm, soapy water.

Taco Seasoning Blend

Spicy, but not too hot, this seasoning mix livens up all your favorite Tex-Mex meals. This recipe is gluten-free.

Yield: 2¹/₂ tablespoons
Prep time: 2 minutes
Serving size: 1 teaspoon
Each serving has:
8 calories
0 g fat
0 g saturated fat
1 g carbohydrates
0 g fiber
0 g protein
235 mg sodium

1 TB. chili powder

¹/₂ TB. ground cumin

¹/₂ tsp. fine sea salt

¹/₂ tsp. freshly ground black pepper

¹/₄ tsp. ground chipotle chili pepper

¹/₄ tsp. crushed red pepper flakes

¹/₄ tsp. garlic powder

¹/₄ tsp. onion powder

¹/₄ tsp. dried oregano

¹/₄ tsp. paprika

1. In a small bowl, combine chili powder, cumin, sea salt, black pepper, chipotle chili pepper, crushed red pepper flakes, garlic powder, onion powder, oregano, and paprika. Stir to blend.

2. Transfer seasoning blend to a glass spice jar with a tight-fitting lid. Store in a cool, dark place.

No-Flour Power _____

Prepared taco seasoning blends sold in envelopes are packaged with sugar and starch. Plus, they're often high in sodium. Experiment with spices and quantities to prepare your own favorite taco seasoning blend at home with no unwanted additives.

Cheese-and-Herb-Stuffed Chicken Breasts

Golden-brown chicken tenderloins enclose a creamy feta and oregano filling with a drizzle of rich chicken glaze for a silky, moist entrée. This recipe is gluten-free if the chicken is gluten-free.

½ cup crumbled feta cheese

1 TB. chopped fresh parsley

½ TB. chopped fresh oregano

⅛ tsp. freshly ground black pepper

1 TB. fat-free milk

12 (about 1 lb.) boneless, skinless chicken breast tenderloins

¼ tsp. fine sea salt

½ cup fat-free, reduced-sodium chicken broth

Yield: 6 servings
Prep time: 10 minutes
Cook time: 21 to 25 minutes
Serving size: 1 stuffed chicken breast plus 2 teaspoons broth
Each serving has:
113 calories
4 g fat
2 g saturated fat
1 g carbohydrates
0 g fiber
20 g protein
321 mg sodium

1. In a small bowl, combine feta cheese, parsley, oregano, and black pepper. Stir to mix. Add milk. Stir until mixture can mound.

2. Spread 1 tablespoon cheese mixture across 6 tenderloins, pressing onto the surface. Arrange 6 tenderloins on top to cover cheese mixture.

3. Heat a large skillet over medium heat. When hot, coat with cooking spray. Add chicken, and sprinkle ⅛ teaspoon sea salt over top. Cook for 5 minutes or until chicken is browned on undersides.

4. Turn chicken, and season with remaining ⅛ teaspoon sea salt. Reduce heat to medium-low. Cover and cook for 8 to 10 minutes or until liquid has released.

5. Pour in broth, and increase heat to medium. Cook, uncovered, for 8 to 10 minutes or until broth is reduced to ¼ cup.

6. To serve, drizzle 2 teaspoons broth reduction over each stuffed chicken breast. Serve hot.

 For Good Measure _____

A reduction is a sauce made simply by simmering or boiling to concentrate the liquid through evaporation. A broth makes a silky sauce. Be sure to choose a reduced-sodium option to keep the reduction from tasting too salty.

Quinoa Turkey Meatloaf

The mild quinoa flavor disappears into the spiced turkey loaf that's topped with a sweetened tomato glaze. This recipe is gluten-free.

Yield: 8 servings
Prep time: 20 to 25 minutes
Cook time: 70 to 75 minutes
Serving size: 1 slice
Each serving has:
228 calories
5 g fat
1 g saturated fat
25 g carbohydrates
2 g fiber
21 g protein
371 mg sodium

1 tsp. extra-virgin olive oil

1 cup diced yellow onions

2 medium cloves garlic, minced

2 TB. dried parsley flakes

1 tsp. fine sea salt

½ tsp. freshly ground black pepper

½ tsp. ground thyme

¼ tsp. cayenne pepper

¼ tsp. dry mustard

½ cup fat-free, plain yogurt

2 large eggs, at room temperature

1.2 lb. ground turkey breast

1 cup cooked quinoa

5 TB. tomato paste

3 TB. water

2 TB. honey

4 tsp. cider vinegar

1. Preheat oven to 350°F.

2. Heat a small skillet over medium heat. When hot, add extra-virgin olive oil. Add onions and garlic. Cook, stirring frequently, for 5 minutes or until golden-brown. Remove from heat.

3. In a large bowl, combine parsley flakes, sea salt, black pepper, thyme, cayenne pepper, dry mustard, yogurt, and eggs. Stir until blended. Add onion mixture, turkey breast, and quinoa. Mix until well combined. Turn into a 9×5×3 nonstick loaf pan and smooth the top. Bake for 45 minutes.

4. Meanwhile, in a small bowl, combine tomato paste, water, honey, and cider vinegar. Stir until blended.

5. Remove meatloaf from the oven and drain, skimming fat from surface as necessary. Run a knife around the edge of the pan. Spread tomato paste mixture over top of meatloaf. Bake for 20 to 25 minutes or until a food thermometer reads 165°F. Let stand for 10 to 15 minutes before cutting into slices to serve.

For Good Measure

If you're concerned about using a metal knife on your nonstick-coated bakeware, opt for a thin, small spatula made of silicone or other pliable material. Many great options for nonscratching utensils are on the market today.

Sprouted Grain–Breaded Pork Chops

Coated with ground garbanzo and fava beans then encrusted in herbed sprouted-grain breadcrumbs, these thick, moist pork chops are a welcome entrée.

¼ cup ground garbanzo and fava beans

¼ tsp. paprika

¼ tsp. fine sea salt

¼ tsp. freshly ground black pepper

2 large eggs, at room temperature

1 cup sprouted-grain breadcrumbs

1 tsp. Italian seasoning

1 tsp. dried parsley flakes

1 lb. 1-inch-thick boneless pork chops, trimmed of fat

Yield: 4 servings
Prep time: 10 minutes
Cook time: 15 minutes
Serving size: 1 pork chop
Each serving has:
196 calories
7 g fat
2 g saturated fat
6 g carbohydrates
2 g fiber
28 g protein
168 mg sodium

1. In a shallow dish, combine ground beans, paprika, sea salt, and black pepper. Stir.

2. In another shallow dish, whisk eggs until lemon-colored.

3. In a third shallow dish, combine breadcrumbs, Italian seasoning, and parsley flakes. Stir.

4. Dredge each pork chop in ground bean mixture to coat, shaking off excess. Dip in egg to coat, allowing excess to drip off. Dredge in breadcrumb mixture to coat completely.

5. Heat a large skillet over medium heat. When hot, coat with cooking spray. Add pork chops to skillet, and cook for 5 minutes on each side or until browned and breading is set. Cover and cook for 5 minutes or until the temperature reads 160°F on a food thermometer.

 For Good Measure

If your pork chops are larger, you may need to cut them to make single-serving sizes. Or, if you want to serve whole pork chops, the breading ingredients are sufficient to coat four larger than 1-pound pork chops.

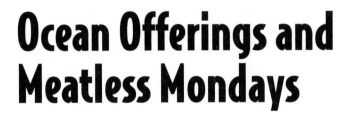

Chapter 14

Ocean Offerings and Meatless Mondays

In This Chapter

- Favorite fish dishes with great flavors
- Seafood entrées featuring crab and shrimp
- Vegetarian choices everyone will savor

When you want to enjoy the tastes of the sea or main dishes picked fresh from the garden, you still need to watch out for hidden flours. Keep the flavor up while you let your guard down and enjoy the recipes offered here.

Coat Check

Even main-dish entrées can be sources of flour in your diet. Flour and flour-based foods—breads, crackers, pretzels, tortilla chips—serve as breadings and coatings. Meats, poultry, fish, seafood, and even vegetables are subject to preparations that involve dredging in flour or coating with flour or flour-based foods. You may even need to keep an eye out for dishes crusted with starchy potato chip crumbs.

Do you have to pass on all these entrées to eat flour-free? Not if you know how this source of flour can be eliminated or substituted. Naturally, the flour alternatives discussed in Chapter 5 are good options. The supermarket's natural foods section or health-food aisle may offer more choices. Look for flour-free versions of crackers, chips, pretzels, and more.

Remember, too, that the ingredients used as coatings can also serve as fillers in your favorite entrées. Beware of dishes such as meatloaf; meatballs; hamburgers; stuffed steak, chicken, pork chops, shrimp, and vegetables; salmon and crab cakes; and other mixed or stuffed recipes.

No-Flour Power

Take advantage of the gluten-free products that are hitting the market. Of course, you'll need to look through the ingredients lists to be certain the foods fit your dietary needs. Still, if an item is marked gluten-free it is also wheat-free.

Macadamia-Crusted Tropical Tilapia

This mild white fish is coated with a subtly sweet, crunchy breading.

¼ cup ground coconut

¼ tsp. fine sea salt

¼ tsp. freshly ground black pepper

⅓ cup fat-free milk

½ cup dry-roasted macadamia nut pieces

¼ cup sprouted-grain breadcrumbs

1 tsp. dried parsley flakes

1 lb. tilapia fillets

Yield: 4 servings
Prep time: 8 minutes
Cook time: 10 minutes
Serving size: 1 fillet
Each serving has:
284 calories
15 g fat
3 g saturated fat
9 g carbohydrates
5 g fiber
28 g protein
232 mg sodium

1. Preheat oven to 425°F.

2. In a shallow dish, combine ground coconut, sea salt, and black pepper.

3. Pour milk into a second shallow dish.

4. Place macadamia nut pieces in a blender. Cover and grind on high speed for 5 seconds or just until nuts are finely ground. Transfer to a third shallow dish and stir in breadcrumbs and parsley flakes.

5. Dredge each tilapia fillet in ground coconut mixture. Dip into milk, wetting both sides. Dredge in macadamia nut mixture to coat.

6. Arrange fillets on a medium nonstick baking sheet coated with cooking spray. Bake for 10 minutes or until fish is opaque and flakes easily with a fork. Cut fillets into 4 equal servings, if needed. Serve hot.

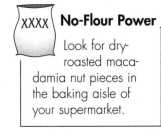

No-Flour Power

Look for dry-roasted macadamia nut pieces in the baking aisle of your supermarket.

Coastline Crab Cakes

Simply seasoned, these crab cakes highlight the flavor of the crabmeat brightened by the tang of fresh lemon juice.

Yield: 3 servings
Prep time: 10 minutes
Cook time: 13 to 15 minutes
Serving size: 2 crab cakes
Each serving has:
162 calories
5 g fat
1 g saturated fat
13 g carbohydrates
2 g fiber
17 g protein
500 mg sodium

2 large eggs, at room temperature

1½ cups sprouted-grain breadcrumbs

¼ cup thinly sliced green onions

¼ cup fresh lemon juice

½ tsp. dry mustard

¼ tsp. fine sea salt

¼ tsp. freshly ground black pepper

1 (6-oz.) pkg. ready-to-eat lump crabmeat

1. Preheat the broiler on high.

2. In a medium bowl, whisk eggs until lemon-colored. Add 1 cup breadcrumbs, green onions, lemon juice, dry mustard, sea salt, and black pepper. Stir until mixed.

3. Flake crabmeat, and add to mixture. Stir to mix. Form mixture into 3-inch patties using ¼ cup for each. Coat each lightly with remaining ½ cup breadcrumbs.

4. Arrange crab cakes on a broiler pan coated with cooking spray. Cook 6 inches from the heating element for 8 to 10 minutes or until browned. Turn and cook for an additional 5 minutes or until browned and crisped.

 No-Flour Power _____

Opt for real lump crabmeat to avoid the starches and sugars found in imitation crabmeat products.

Coconut-Coated Shrimp

Succulent super-sized shrimp shine in a lightly toasted coating of coconut that benefits from its natural sweetness. This recipe is gluten-free.

¼ **cup plus 1 TB. ground coconut**

⅛ **tsp. fine sea salt**

⅛ **tsp. cayenne pepper**

⅔ **cup fat-free milk**

½ **cup unsweetened medium-cut, flaked coconut**

1 (14-oz.) **pkg. peeled, deveined, tail-on, jumbo uncooked shrimp**

Yield: 4 servings
Prep time: 25 minutes
Cook time: 8 minutes
Serving size: 6 shrimp
Each serving has:
295 calories
14 g fat
11 g saturated fat
16 g carbohydrates
7 g fiber
26 g protein
245 mg sodium

1. Preheat the oven to 400°F.

2. In a shallow dish, combine ¼ cup ground coconut, sea salt, and cayenne pepper. Stir.

3. Pour milk into a small bowl.

4. In another shallow dish, combine flaked coconut and 1 tablespoon ground coconut. Stir.

5. Holding each shrimp by the tail, dredge shrimp in seasoned ground coconut, shaking off excess. Dip in milk to coat, allowing excess to drip off. Dredge in flaked coconut mixture to coat evenly.

6. Arrange coated shrimp in a single layer on a large nonstick baking sheet coated with cooking spray. Bake for 4 minutes. Turn shrimp, and bake for 4 more minutes or until shrimp are done, opaque and pink, and coconut is lightly toasted.

 For Good Measure

Shrimp are gray-colored and translucent when raw. When cooked, shrimp become opaque and a lovely shade of pink.

Broiled Salmon with Dilled Tartar Sauce

This lightly lemon- and garlic-flavored fish is accompanied by a fresh-made, dill-infused tartar sauce with just enough "tart" to tingle the taste buds. This recipe is gluten-free.

Yield: 4 servings
Prep time: 2 minutes
Cook time: 10 minutes
Chill time: 30 minutes
Serving size: 1 piece salmon plus 1½ table-spoons tartar sauce

Each serving has:
313 calories
23 g fat
4 g saturated fat
2 g carbohydrates
1 g fiber
24 g protein
90 mg sodium

⅓ cup Fresh-Made Mayonnaise (see Chapter 10)

2 TB. chopped fresh dill

1 TB. minced green onions

2 tsp. fresh lemon juice

Pinch fine sea salt

Pinch freshly ground black pepper

1 lb. 1-inch-thick skinless salmon fillet

¼ tsp. garlic powder

4 thin slices lemon

1. To make Dilled Tartar Sauce, combine Fresh-Made Mayonnaise, dill, green onions, lemon juice, sea salt, and black pepper in a small bowl. Stir to blend. Cover and chill for at least 30 minutes before serving. Use within 5 days.

2. Meanwhile, preheat the broiler on high with the oven rack positioned to broil 6 inches from the heating element.

3. Arrange salmon on a broiler pan coated with cooking spray. Broil for 5 minutes. Sprinkle garlic powder over salmon. Top with lemon slices, spacing evenly. Broil for 5 more minutes or until salmon is opaque and flakes easily with a fork.

4. Cut salmon into 4 equal pieces. Serve with Dilled Tartar Sauce.

No-Flour Power

If you love salmon but are concerned about the reported high mercury levels in this fish, opt for wild salmon instead of farm-raised options. Wild-caught salmon boasts lower mercury contamination. Wild salmon will be marked as such and is available both fresh and frozen.

Easy Eggplant Parmigiana Casserole

Tender eggplant slices are baked in tomato sauce and cheeses for a clean, fresh taste without the grease and breading. This recipe is gluten-free.

1 medium eggplant

2¾ cups No-Cook Italian Pasta Sauce (recipe later in this chapter)

1 cup shredded part-skim, low-moisture mozzarella cheese

¼ cup shredded Parmesan cheese

Yield: 8 servings
Prep time: 15 minutes
Cook time: 1 hour
Serving size: 2 eggplant slices plus ⅓ cup sauce
Each serving has:
135 calories
6 g fat
5 g saturated fat
12 g carbohydrates
4 g fiber
8 g protein
244 mg sodium

1. Preheat the oven to 350°F.

2. Trim stem and blossom ends from eggplant, and discard. Cut eggplant into 16 ½-inch slices.

3. Spread ½ cup pasta sauce in the bottom of a 13×9×2 baking dish. Layer half of eggplant slices on top, cutting to fit, if needed. Spoon half of remaining pasta sauce over top. Sprinkle ½ cup mozzarella cheese over top. Layer remaining eggplant slices on top. Spoon remaining pasta sauce over eggplant. Cover tightly with foil and bake for 55 minutes or until eggplant is tender.

4. Carefully uncover casserole. Sprinkle remaining ½ cup mozzarella cheese and Parmesan cheese over all. Bake, uncovered, for 5 minutes or until cheeses are melted. Let stand for 5 minutes before serving. Serve with cooked brown rice spaghetti pasta, if desired.

Starch Guard

Take care when removing the covers from baked items. Although virtually invisible, steam can cause burns.

No-Cook Italian Pasta Sauce

The tangy taste of tomatoes is smoothed by extra-virgin olive oil and honey with the seasoning of garlic and fresh herbs in this sauce. This recipe is gluten-free.

Yield: 2¾ cups
Prep time: 5 minutes
Serving size: ¼ cup
Each serving has:
43 calories
2 g fat
0 g saturated fat
5 g carbohydrates
1 g fiber
1 g protein
82 mg sodium

1 (14.5-oz.) can petite-cut diced tomatoes, undrained

1 (6-oz.) can tomato paste

½ cup water

1½ TB. extra-virgin olive oil

1 tsp. honey

1 large clove garlic, minced

2 TB. chopped fresh basil

2 TB. chopped fresh oregano

In a medium bowl, combine tomatoes, tomato paste, water, extra-virgin olive oil, honey, garlic, basil, and oregano. Stir until well blended. Use as you would a jarred spaghetti sauce in recipes.

XXXX **No-Flour Power**

When fresh herbs are unavailable, you can substitute dried herbs at a 3:1 ratio. For each tablespoon of a fresh herb, substitute 1 teaspoon dried. Then, adjust seasonings to taste, as usual.

Moroccan Quinoa-Stuffed Bell Peppers

This savory quinoa filling is studded with the sweetness of sun-dried tomatoes, golden raisins, and cinnamon in sweet bell pepper halves. This recipe is gluten-free.

4 sun-dried tomato halves	**¾ cup cooked quinoa**
¼ cup boiling water	**3 TB. golden raisins**
3 TB. pine nuts	**⅛ tsp. freshly ground black pepper**
1 tsp. extra-virgin olive oil	
⅓ cup diced yellow onions	**⅛ tsp. ground cinnamon**
1 medium clove garlic, minced	**1 large orange bell pepper**

Yield: 2 servings
Prep time: 15 minutes
Cook time: 26 minutes
Serving size: 1 bell pepper half
Each serving has:
450 calories
13 g fat
2 g saturated fat
71 g carbohydrates
8 g fiber
12 g protein
184 mg sodium

1. Preheat the oven to 375°F.

2. Place sun-dried tomatoes in a small bowl. Pour boiling water over top. Let stand for 5 minutes or until softened. Remove from water and finely chop.

3. Meanwhile, in a small skillet over medium heat, toast pine nuts for 3 minutes or until golden-brown, shaking the skillet occasionally to prevent burning. Remove pine nuts to a medium bowl.

4. In the same small skillet over medium heat, add extra-virgin olive oil. Add onions and sauté, stirring frequently, for 2 minutes or until softened. Add garlic. Cook and stir for 1 minute or until golden. Turn mixture into pine nuts.

5. Add quinoa, sun-dried tomatoes, golden raisins, black pepper, and cinnamon to pine nut mixture. Stir to mix.

6. Cut orange bell pepper in half. Remove seeds and ribs. Spoon pine nut mixture into bell pepper halves. Arrange in a small baking dish coated with cooking spray. Bake for 20 minutes or until bell peppers are tender-crisp and filling is golden-brown. Serve hot.

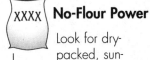

No-Flour Power

Look for dry-packed, sun-dried tomatoes in your grocer's produce department.

Savory Dinner Pancakes with Green Onion Salsa

Topped with a fresh, chunky salsa, these filling pancakes are lightly spiced with cumin. This recipe is gluten-free.

Yield: 5 servings
Prep time: 12 minutes
Cook time: 4 minutes per batch
Serving size: 2 pancakes plus 2 tablespoons salsa
Each serving has:
200 calories
4 g fat
0 g saturated fat
30 g carbohydrates
10 g fiber
11 g protein
474 mg sodium

⅓ cup seeded, diced tomatoes

⅓ cup sliced green onions

1 TB. fresh lime juice

2 tsp. chopped fresh cilantro

2 cups ground garbanzo and fava beans

1 tsp. ground cumin

1 tsp. fine sea salt

1 large egg, at room temperature

1½ cups water

1. In a small bowl, combine tomatoes, green onions, lime juice, and cilantro. Stir to mix. Set aside while you prepare pancakes.

2. In a large bowl, combine ground beans, cumin, and sea salt. Stir to mix.

3. In a small bowl, whisk egg until lemon-colored. Add to dry ingredients. While whisking, gradually pour in water, and continue whisking until batter is smooth.

4. Heat a large nonstick skillet over medium heat. When hot, pour in ¼ cup batter for each pancake. Cook for 2 minutes or until tops are bubbly and edges are dry. Turn and cook on the other side for 2 minutes or until undersides are golden-brown. Repeat with remaining batter, keeping cooked pancakes in a warm oven. To serve, spoon salsa over pancakes.

For Good Measure

Preparing pancakes is easy if you remain patient. Pancakes can be flipped only once—but they let you know when they're ready. Watch for small bubbles on the surface, and check for the outer edges to look dry. Then flip and finish.

Mushroom, Almond, and Brown Rice Stuffed Zucchini

Whether presented as a vegetarian entrée or a single-serve side dish, these scrumptious baked zucchini boats are loaded with a delectable mix of veggies, grains, nuts, and seasonings. This recipe is gluten-free.

4 (7- to 8-inch) zucchini	1 cup ground almond meal
½ TB. extra-virgin olive oil	3 TB. fresh lemon juice
1½ cups minced yellow onions	2 TB. chopped fresh chives
3 cups very finely chopped white button mushrooms	¼ tsp. cayenne pepper
	¼ tsp. fine sea salt
4 large cloves garlic, minced	⅛ tsp. freshly ground black pepper
1 cup cooked, long-grain brown rice	

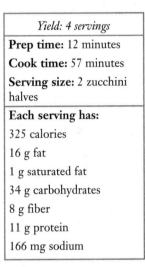

Yield: 4 servings
Prep time: 12 minutes
Cook time: 57 minutes
Serving size: 2 zucchini halves
Each serving has:
325 calories
16 g fat
1 g saturated fat
34 g carbohydrates
8 g fiber
11 g protein
166 mg sodium

1. Preheat the oven to 350°F.

2. Trim ends from zucchini and discard. Cut zucchini in half lengthwise. Using a small spoon, remove the seeds and pulp, leaving about a ¼-inch margin of zucchini flesh. Finely chop removed zucchini and set aside. Arrange zucchini halves in a 13×9×2 baking dish.

3. Heat a large skillet over medium heat. When hot, add extra-virgin olive oil. Add onions and cook, stirring occasionally, for 5 minutes or until softened. Add finely chopped zucchini and mushrooms. Cook, stirring occasionally, for 10 minutes or until vegetables are tender. Add garlic and cook, stirring occasionally, for 2 minutes.

4. In a large bowl, combine brown rice, ground almond meal, onion mixture, lemon juice, chives, cayenne pepper, sea salt, and black pepper. Stir until mixed. Spoon into hollows of zucchini halves. Bake for 40 minutes or until zucchini halves are tender.

For Good Measure

Knowing how to interpret a recipe's ingredients list will help ensure a successful dish. A call for "1 cup diced onions" is different than "1 small onion, diced." The former instructs you to measure the onions after you've diced them; the latter calls for a small onion that you then prepare by dicing.

Plenty of Pasta-bilities

In This Chapter

- ◆ Flourless alternative pasta dishes
- ◆ Pre-packaged brown rice, quinoa, corn, and konjac pasta shapes
- ◆ Edible and delectable pasta stand-ins

Pasta makes for a filling meal with endless combinations of sauces, cheeses, vegetables, and meats—but it's made of wheat flour. Eating flour-free means you need to stock your kitchen with healthful alternatives.

A Twist on Twirling

Traditional flour pastas can be replaced by prepackaged alternatives or creative edible substitutes. As always, check ingredients lists to be certain the prepared products fit your dietary needs.

Brown rice pasta can be purchased in numerous traditional pasta shapes, including fusilli, rotini, elbow macaroni, spaghetti, linguini, shells, and more. Brown rice pastas will remind you of dried traditional flour pastas, but they are best eaten immediately after cooking, as they tend to get mushy upon sitting.

Corn pasta may be plain or combined with vegetable flavors. You'll find plenty of shapes—spaghetti, rotini, radiatore, shells, and others.

Konjac noodles, sold in several shapes, are packaged in water. Konjac is a dietary fiber which has a texture that is chewy and elastic.

Quinoa pasta is made with a blend of quinoa and corn grains. You can choose from several shapes, including shells and elbow macaroni. Quinoa pastas have a slightly chewy texture.

Spaghetti squash is a hard-shelled winter squash with a yellow-beige peel. When cooked, the flesh of this squash naturally shreds into spaghettilike strands. Top it with your favorite sauces.

Zucchini and eggplant, when sliced lengthwise, can be layered like lasagna noodles.

Spaghetti Squash with Fresh Tomato Sauce

This mild-flavored winter squash serves as a bed for the vinegar-brightened tomato and basil no-cook sauce. This recipe is gluten-free.

2 cups seeded, diced tomatoes

½ cup diced yellow or sweet onions

¼ cup chopped fresh basil

2 TB. red wine vinegar

1 TB. extra-virgin olive oil

½ tsp. agave nectar

1 (9-inch) spaghetti squash

Yield: 4 servings
Prep time: 18 minutes
Cook time: 1 hour
Serving size: 1 cup squash plus ½ cup sauce
Each serving has:
103 calories
4 g fat
1 g saturated fat
15 g carbohydrates
3 g fiber
2 g protein
13 mg sodium

1. Preheat oven to 375°F.

2. In a medium bowl, combine tomatoes, onions, basil, red wine vinegar, extra-virgin olive oil, and agave nectar. Stir to mix. Let stand at room temperature while spaghetti squash cooks.

3. With a large, sharp knife, cut spaghetti squash in half lengthwise. Using a large spoon, scoop out strings and seeds; discard.

4. Place spaghetti squash halves cut side down in a 13×9×2 or larger baking dish. Add ½ inch water to the bottom of the dish. Bake for 1 hour or until tender.

5. Carefully remove spaghetti squash halves from baking dish. Using the tines of a fork, scrape the flesh out of the shell, pulling into long, spaghettilike strands. Drain as needed.

6. To serve, make a bed of spaghetti squash, and cover with fresh tomato sauce. If desired, sprinkle shredded Parmesan cheese to taste over top.

For Good Measure

The flesh of the spaghetti squash lends itself as a pasta substitute for both salads and entrées.

Three Cheese White Zucchini Lasagna

All the traditional cheesy taste of lasagna is stacked here between zucchini slices in a creamy Parmesan sauce. This recipe is gluten-free.

Yield: 6 servings
Prep time: 10 minutes
Cook time: 1 hour 15 minutes
Serving size: 2⅝×4-inch square
Each serving has:
254 calories
15 g fat
9 g saturated fat
12 g carbohydrates
1 g fiber
17 g protein
377 mg sodium

3 TB. unsalted butter

3 TB. stone-ground brown rice

⅛ tsp. fine sea salt

⅛ tsp. freshly ground black pepper

1½ cups fat-free milk

½ cup plus 2 TB. shredded Parmesan cheese

1 cup part-skim ricotta cheese

¾ cup shredded part-skim, low-moisture mozzarella cheese

1 large egg

½ tsp. dried basil

½ tsp. dried oregano

2 (8-inch) zucchini

1. Preheat oven to 350°F.

2. Melt butter in a medium saucepan over medium heat. When butter is bubbly, whisk in stone-ground brown rice, sea salt, and black pepper until moistened. Gradually whisk in milk until smooth. Continue whisking for 5 minutes or until mixture begins to thicken. Turn off heat. Stir in ½ cup Parmesan cheese until smooth. Remove from heat.

3. In a medium bowl, combine ricotta cheese, mozzarella cheese, egg, basil, and oregano. Stir until blended.

4. Trim ends from zucchini and discard. Cut zucchini lengthwise into 9 slices, about ¼-inch thick.

5. Spread a thin layer of Parmesan sauce across the bottom of an 8×8×2 baking dish. Layer 3 zucchini slices, ⅓ of ricotta cheese mixture, and ¼ of remaining Parmesan sauce. Repeat layering twice. Spread remaining Parmesan sauce over top.

6. Bake, covered, for 60 minutes. Uncover and sprinkle 2 tablespoons Parmesan cheese over top. Bake for an additional 5 to 10 minutes or until top is golden-brown. Let stand for 15 minutes before serving.

Variation: Add a thin layer of vegetables atop the ricotta cheese mixture. Try shredded carrots, sliced mushrooms, chopped spinach, or any other favorites.

For Good Measure

Eggs are packed in their cartons, broad ends up, because it keeps the yolks centered.

Summer-Style Puttanesca Pasta

An easy-to-prepare meal, this no-cook sauce is a hot and tangy topper for the bed of brown rice penne pasta. This recipe is gluten-free.

2 cups chopped tomatoes

¾ cup coarsely chopped kalamata olives

¼ cup drained capers

¼ cup fresh oregano leaves

2 TB. extra-virgin olive oil

6 medium cloves garlic, minced

1 tsp. crushed red pepper flakes

¼ tsp. freshly ground black pepper

8 oz. (about 2 cups) uncooked brown rice penne pasta

½ cup chopped fresh parsley

½ cup shredded Parmesan cheese

Yield: 6 servings
Prep time: 5 minutes
Cook time: 16 minutes
Serving size: 1 cup plus 4 teaspoons each parsley and Parmesan cheese
Each serving has:
251 calories
10 g fat
2 g saturated fat
35 g carbohydrates
4 g fiber
6 g protein
411 mg sodium

1. In a large serving bowl, combine tomatoes, kalamata olives, capers, oregano leaves, extra-virgin olive oil, garlic, crushed red pepper flakes, and black pepper. Stir to distribute evenly. Set aside at room temperature.

2. Prepare brown rice penne pasta according to the package directions, omitting salt. Rinse and drain. Add pasta to tomato mixture, and stir to coat evenly.

3. Top each serving with 2 tablespoons parsley and 2 tablespoons shredded Parmesan cheese.

Variation: You may seed the tomatoes, if preferred.

No-Flour Power

To remove the papery covering from a garlic clove easily, place the clove on a cutting board or other hard, flat surface. Lay the wide blade of a knife, such as a butcher's knife, horizontally on top of the clove (sharp edge away from you). Carefully pound the heel of your hand on the knife blade. The peel will release.

Garlicky Fusilli with Ham, Greens, and Walnuts

Twirling strands of brown rice pasta are enlivened here with a garlic-flavored olive oil, lemon-kissed kale, meaty walnuts, and diced ham. This recipe is gluten-free.

Yield: 7 servings
Prep time: 5 minutes
Cook time: 17 to 20 minutes
Serving size: 1 cup
Each serving has:
230 calories
9 g fat
1 g saturated fat
30 g carbohydrates
2 g fiber
7 g protein
150 mg sodium

4 cups packed torn kale

½ cup hot water, or as needed

1 tsp. fresh lemon juice

4 oz. (about ¾ cup) diced natural Black Forest deli ham

½ cup chopped walnuts

3 medium cloves garlic, minced

⅛ tsp. fine sea salt

⅛ tsp. freshly ground black pepper

2½ cups uncooked brown rice fusilli pasta

1 TB. extra-virgin olive oil

1. Wash kale, and place, along with the water that clings to the leaves, in an extra-large skillet over medium heat. Cook, stirring often, for 12 to 15 minutes or until wilted. Add hot water a little at a time as needed to keep the skillet from cooking dry.

2. When kale is wilted and skillet is nearly dry, sprinkle on lemon juice. Add ham, walnuts, garlic, sea salt, and black pepper. Cook, stirring occasionally, for 5 minutes or until ham starts to brown.

3. Meanwhile, prepare brown rice fusilli pasta according to the package directions, omitting any salt or oil suggested. Rinse and drain well. Transfer pasta to a large serving bowl. Add extra-virgin olive oil, and stir to coat. Add kale mixture to pasta, and stir to distribute evenly. Serve hot with shredded Parmesan cheese, if desired.

No-Flour Power _____

Deli hams are processed meats, so look for natural selections without additives, preservatives, and starches. You can find products without nitrates and nitrites, those cured with sea salt, and hams cured with minimal sugar. Uncured hams are also available.

Cincinnati Turkey Chili with Beans

Turn a mildly spiced pot of turkey chili into a meal with this bed of al dente brown rice spaghetti pasta and a sprinkling of raw onions and melty cheddar cheese. This recipe is gluten-free.

1 lb. ground turkey breast	**1½ cups water**
½ cup plus ¾ cup diced yellow onions	**2 cups cooked pinto beans**
½ cup finely chopped green bell peppers	**1 TB. chili powder**
1 medium clove garlic, minced	**½ tsp. dried oregano**
	½ tsp. fine sea salt
1 (14.5-oz.) can petite-cut diced tomatoes, undrained	**⅛ tsp. ground ginger**
1 (6-oz.) can tomato paste	**12 oz. uncooked brown rice spaghetti pasta**
	¾ cup shredded cheddar cheese

Yield: 12 servings
Prep time: 5 minutes
Cook time: 1 hour 40 minutes
Serving size: ½ heaping cup chili with ½ cup pasta
Each serving has:
246 calories
5 g fat
2 g saturated fat
35 g carbohydrates
5 g fiber
16 g protein
254 mg sodium

1. In a large saucepan, combine turkey breast, ½ cup diced onions, green bell peppers, and garlic. Cook over medium heat for 10 minutes or until turkey is browned; stir to break up turkey into small pieces.

2. Add diced tomatoes, tomato paste, and water. Stir to blend. Add pinto beans, chili powder, oregano, sea salt, and ginger. Stir. Bring to a boil.

3. Reduce heat to low. Cover and simmer for 1½ hours.

4. Meanwhile, cook pasta according to the package directions. Rinse and drain.

5. Line serving plates with pasta. Top with chili. Sprinkle 2 tablespoons diced onions and 2 tablespoons cheese over each serving. Serve hot.

No-Flour Power

Save on added fat and sodium by cooking all your pasta substitutes plain. Package directions may call for adding oil or salt to the cooking water, but these suggestions are optional—as well as unnecessary. Simply stirring your pasta occasionally while cooking in a roomy pot will keep it from sticking.

Kielbasa and Kraut Caraway Noodle Casserole

The bite of sauerkraut seasoned with caraway seeds and the meaty texture of kielbasa complement creamy corn noodles in this hearty dish. This recipe is gluten-free.

Yield: 6 servings
Prep time: 8 minutes
Cook time: 36 minutes
Serving size: 1 cup
Each serving has:
273 calories
13 g fat
5 g saturated fat
30 g carbohydrates
1 g fiber
9 g protein
560 mg sodium

6 oz. corn vegetable radiatore noodles

1⅛ cups Versatile Flourless White Sauce (see Chapter 16)

8 oz. natural Polish kielbasa, thinly sliced

1½ cups Polish sauerkraut with caraway seeds, drained

¼ cup minced yellow onions

1. Preheat oven to 350°F.

2. Cook corn noodles according to the package directions until al dente. Rinse and drain.

3. In a large bowl, combine corn noodles, Versatile Flourless White Sauce, kielbasa, sauerkraut, and onions. Stir to mix.

4. Turn mixture into an 8×8×2 baking dish coated with cooking spray. Bake, uncovered, for 30 minutes or until bubbly and heated through. Serve hot.

For Good Measure

Kielbasa is a processed meat product that can vary greatly from brand to brand and style to style. Look for natural products without preservatives and added nitrates and nitrites. Read the ingredients lists and nutrition data boxes for the least amount of sugars and salts used in processing.

Tomato and Clam Konjac Linguini

A tomato-tinged butter sauce with a touch of heat coats these clams and linguini for a tasty, textured pasta dish. This recipe is gluten-free.

3 TB. unsalted butter

2 medium cloves garlic, minced

¼ tsp. crushed red pepper flakes, or more to taste

1 cup seeded, diced tomatoes

¼ cup shredded Parmesan cheese

¼ cup chopped fresh parsley

½ tsp. fine sea salt

⅛ tsp. freshly ground black pepper

2 (6½-oz.) cans chopped clams

1 (9-oz.) pkg. konjac shirataki linguini noodles

Yield: 3 servings
Prep time: 3 minutes
Cook time: 7 minutes
Serving size: 1 cup
Each serving has:
211 calories
14 g fat
8 g saturated fat
11 g carbohydrates
4 g fiber
12 g protein
589 mg sodium

1. In a large skillet over medium heat, melt butter. Add garlic and crushed red pepper flakes. Cook and stir for 1 minute. Add tomatoes, Parmesan cheese, parsley, sea salt, and black pepper. Cook, stirring frequently, for 3 minutes.

2. Rinse and drain clams and konjac shirataki linguini noodles. Add to tomato mixture. Cook and stir for 1 minute or until heated through. Serve immediately.

No-Flour Power

Canned food items vary widely from brand to brand. The only sure way to know what you're eating is to read the ingredients lists. Two cans sitting side by side on the shelf may affect your health differently. For instance, some clams may be packed with sugars. Read those food labels.

Tuna and Brown Rice Noodle Casserole

This classic creamy tuna casserole is enhanced with the heartiness of chopped mushrooms. This recipe is gluten-free.

Yield: 5 servings
Prep time: 4 minutes
Cook time: 52 minutes
Serving size: 1 cup
Each serving has:
189 calories
7 g fat
3 g saturated fat
20 g carbohydrates
2 g fiber
12 g protein
234 mg sodium

1¾ cups uncooked brown rice elbow macaroni pasta

1 tsp. extra-virgin olive oil

1 cup finely chopped white button mushrooms

2 TB. minced green bell peppers

2 TB. minced yellow onions

1 (6.4-oz.) pkg. light tuna packed in water

1⅛ cups Versatile Flourless White Sauce (see Chapter 16)

1. Preheat oven to 350°F.

2. Prepare pasta according to the package directions until al dente. Rinse and drain.

3. Meanwhile, heat a small skillet over medium heat. When hot, add extra-virgin olive oil. Add mushrooms, green bell peppers, and onions. Cook, stirring frequently, for 5 minutes or until vegetables are softened.

4. In a large bowl, combine pasta, mushroom mixture, tuna, and Versatile Flourless White Sauce. Stir to mix. Spoon into a 1-quart baking dish coated with cooking spray. Bake, uncovered, for 30 minutes or until heated through and the top is browned.

No-Flour Power _____

When recipes call for alternative pastas to be prepared according to the package directions, you can use your favorite pasta substitute, be it brown rice, quinoa, corn, or another style of flourless noodles.

Sun-Dried Tomato and Artichoke Heart Quinoa Pasta

Crushed red pepper flakes kick up the heat in this creamy pasta dish accented with the intense taste of sun-dried tomatoes and velvety artichoke hearts. This recipe is gluten-free.

8 sun-dried tomato halves

1 cup boiling water

1½ cups quinoa elbow or shells pasta

2 tsp. extra-virgin olive oil

3 medium cloves garlic, minced

1 tsp. crushed red pepper flakes or less to taste

1 (13¾-oz.) can quartered artichoke hearts in brine, drained

1 TB. ground garbanzo and fava beans

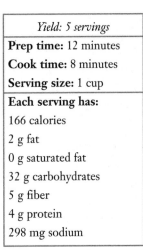

Yield: 5 servings		
Prep time: 12 minutes		
Cook time: 8 minutes		
Serving size: 1 cup		
Each serving has:		
166 calories		
2 g fat		
0 g saturated fat		
32 g carbohydrates		
5 g fiber		
4 g protein		
298 mg sodium		

1. Place sun-dried tomato halves in a small glass bowl. Pour boiling water over top, and let stand for 10 minutes or until softened. Remove tomato halves, allowing excess water to drain off. Cut tomato halves into thin strips. Reserve water.

2. Meanwhile, prepare quinoa pasta according to the package directions until al dente. Rinse and drain.

3. Heat extra-virgin olive oil in a large skillet over medium heat. Stir in garlic and crushed red pepper flakes. Cook and stir for 1 to 2 minutes or until garlic is golden.

4. Stir in artichoke hearts and tomato strips. Reduce heat to medium-low. Cook and stir for 1 to 2 minutes. Whisk ground beans into cooled reserved water, and add to the skillet. Increase heat to medium and bring mixture to a simmer. Cook for 2 minutes, stirring occasionally.

5. Add quinoa pasta to artichoke heart mixture in the skillet, stirring to combine. Heat through, and serve hot. Sprinkle grated Parmesan cheese over individual servings, if desired.

For Good Measure

Dry-packed sun-dried tomatoes will keep indefinitely if stored in an airtight container in a cool, dry place.

Chapter 16

On-the-Side Elections

In This Chapter

- ◆ Filling side dishes using flourless pasta substitutes
- ◆ Tasty trimmings made with flourless bread and flour alternatives
- ◆ Savory sauces and gravy thickened the flour-free way

An entrée presented all by itself on a dinner plate doesn't satisfy your desire for a good meal. You want tasty, yet flour-free accompaniments to round out your eating experiences. This chapter addresses that need.

Choice Cooking Oils

Cooking oils are a pantry staple. Some, such as walnut oil and sesame seed oil, infuse flavor into the dish. Others are practical, such as corn oil and safflower oils that get the cooking done. But another consideration when choosing a cooking oil is its *smoke point*. Heating any oil to its smoke point can potentially change it into a toxic substance. If your cooking oil oxidizes and begins to smoke while heating, discard it.

Words to Digest _____

Smoke point denotes the temperature at which a cooking oil begins to smolder. Heating oil to the smoke point breaks it down, leaving it unfit to eat.

The cooking oil most called for in this cookbook is extra-virgin olive oil because of its monounsaturated, heart-healthy properties. The smoke point is relatively low, though, so don't heat it higher than 375°F (or about 320°F if it's unrefined). If you need a high-heat cooking oil, opt for peanut oil, sunflower oil, or extra-light olive oil—each with a smoke point around 450°F.

Golden-Topped Quinoa Shells and Cheese

This version of mac-and-cheese is sure to please with its super-grain quinoa pasta shells coated in a creamy, tangy cheddar sauce. This recipe is gluten-free.

1 (8-oz.) pkg. quinoa shells pasta	**2½ cups prepared Cheddar Cheese Sauce (recipe later in this chapter)**

1. Preheat oven to 375°F.

2. Cook pasta according to the package directions until al dente, omitting any salt or oil suggested. Rinse and drain. Turn into a 1-quart baking dish coated with cooking spray.

3. Add Cheddar Cheese Sauce, and stir to coat evenly. Bake, uncovered, for 15 minutes or until top is golden and mixture is heated through. Serve hot.

Yield: 10 servings
Prep time: 4 minutes
Cook time: 28 minutes
Serving size: ½ cup
Each serving has:
183 calories
7 g fat
4 g saturated fat
24 g carbohydrates
2 g fiber
5 g protein
158 mg sodium

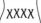

No-Flour Power

Quinoa pasta and other pasta substitutes usually benefit from being rinsed during the draining process. It keeps the pasta from clumping.

Broccoli Cheese and Quinoa Casserole

Rich and cheesy with a tang of sharp cheddar, this broccoli bake will please your pickiest veggie-haters. This recipe is gluten-free.

Yield: 5 servings
Prep time: 3 minutes
Cook time: 34 minutes
Serving size: ½ cup
Each serving has:
339 calories
20 g fat
12 g saturated fat
27 g carbohydrates
3 g fiber
12 g protein
294 mg sodium

2 cups chopped fresh broccoli

½ cup diced yellow onions

1 cup cooked quinoa

1 cup shredded sharp cheddar cheese

¼ cup unsalted butter, cut in small pieces

¼ tsp. fine sea salt

¼ tsp. freshly ground black pepper

1. Preheat oven to 350°F.

2. Combine broccoli and onions in a steamer basket over 1 inch of water. Cover and bring to a boil over high heat. Reduce heat to medium, and steam for 5 minutes or until vegetables are tender-crisp.

3. In a medium bowl, combine broccoli mixture, quinoa, cheese, butter, sea salt, and black pepper. Stir to mix.

4. Spoon mixture into a 1-quart baking dish coated with cooking spray. Bake uncovered for 25 minutes or until bubbly. Serve hot.

XXXX No-Flour Power _____

To measure the cooked quinoa, press it lightly into the measuring cup, fluffing as you stir it into the mixture.

Hungarian Cabbage and Noodles

Butter-glazed fusilli and fried cabbage are combined with a touch of garlic for this simple side dish. This recipe is gluten-free.

2½ cups uncooked brown rice fusilli pasta

3 TB. unsalted butter

6 cups coarsely chopped green cabbage

1 tsp. fine sea salt

1 medium clove garlic, minced

¼ tsp. freshly ground black pepper

Yield: 8 servings
Prep time: 3 minutes
Cook time: 25 minutes
Serving size: ¾ cup
Each serving has:
159 calories
5 g fat
3 g saturated fat
25 g carbohydrates
3 g fiber
3 g protein
293 mg sodium

1. Cook pasta according to the package directions until al dente. Rinse and drain.

2. In an extra-large skillet over medium heat, melt 2 tablespoons butter. Add cabbage and sea salt. Cook, stirring frequently, for 12 minutes or until cabbage is wilted and starting to brown.

3. Reduce heat to low. Add garlic, black pepper, pasta, and 1 tablespoon butter. Cook and stir for 3 minutes or until butter is melted. Cook, stirring occasionally, for 5 minutes to heat through. Serve hot.

Variation: Substitute an equal amount of broken fettuccini noodles, brown rice, corn, or your preferred alternative pasta.

No-Flour Power

For the longest shelf life, keep the garlic bulb intact—papery covering, root end, and all—removing each clove as needed. If you accidentally break off a clove, use it within one week.

Apricot and Walnut Sprouted-Grain Dressing

This toasty flourless bread dressing offers the crunch of walnuts and sesame seeds along with a touch of sweetness with chopped dried apricots and cinnamon.

Yield: 10 servings
Prep time: 18 minutes
Cook time: 30 minutes
Serving size: ½ cup
Each serving has:
134 calories
6 g fat
2 g saturated fat
17 g carbohydrates
4 g fiber
4 g protein
53 mg sodium

⅔ cup dried apricots

1 cup boiling water

2 TB. unsalted butter

⅔ cup diced yellow onions

½ cup thinly sliced celery

5 cups sprouted-grain bread cubes

⅓ cup chopped walnuts

2 TB. toasted sesame seeds

½ tsp. ground cinnamon

⅛ tsp. freshly ground black pepper

1. Preheat oven to 350°F.

2. In a small bowl, soak apricots in boiling water for 15 minutes. Drain, reserving water. Chop apricots.

3. Meanwhile, melt butter in a small skillet over medium heat. Add onions and celery. Cook, stirring occasionally, for 7 minutes or until golden. Remove from heat to cool slightly.

4. In a large bowl, pour reserved water over bread cubes, and stir. Add chopped apricots, onion mixture, walnuts, sesame seeds, cinnamon, and black pepper. Stir to mix.

5. Spoon mixture into an 8×8×2 baking pan coated with cooking spray. Bake, uncovered, for 30 minutes or until top is toasted. Serve hot.

Variation: For a moist dressing, add additional water or fat-free, reduced-sodium chicken broth or vegetable broth to taste.

XXXX No-Flour Power

You'll need about 6 slices of stale sprouted-grain bread to yield 5 cups bread cubes. Tear bread slices into small, bite-size cubes.

Summer Squash Gratin

A creamy and delicious serving of summer's best bounty is mingled with Parmesan cheese and buttered breadcrumbs in this dish.

1 tsp. extra-virgin olive oil

1½ cups thinly sliced yellow squash

1½ cups thinly sliced zucchini

½ cup thinly sliced yellow onions

½ cup fat-free milk

1 TB. stone-ground brown rice

¼ cup shredded Parmesan cheese

¼ tsp. fine sea salt

¼ tsp. freshly ground black pepper

¼ cup sprouted-grain bread-crumbs

1 TB. unsalted butter, cut in small pieces

Yield: 5 servings
Prep time: 5 minutes
Cook time: 27 minutes
Serving size: ½ cup
Each serving has:
88 calories
5 g fat
2 g saturated fat
8 g carbohydrates
2 g fiber
4 g protein
200 mg sodium

1. Preheat oven to 350°F.

2. Heat a large skillet over medium heat. When hot, add extra-virgin olive oil. Add yellow squash, zucchini, and onions. Cook, stirring frequently, for 7 minutes or until softened.

3. Turn half of squash mixture into an 8×2 round baking dish coated with cooking spray. Pour half of milk over squash mixture. Sprinkle half of stone-ground brown rice evenly over top. Sprinkle on half of Parmesan cheese, half of sea salt, and half of black pepper. Repeat layering.

4. Sprinkle breadcrumbs evenly across the top. Dot with butter.

5. Bake uncovered for 20 minutes or until bubbly. Let stand for 5 minutes before serving. Serve hot.

For Good Measure

Parmesan is a hard cheese, so if you open your chunk of cheese and suspect a mold spot, cut a 1-inch margin around the area. The remaining cheese is still safe to eat. By wrapping and then storing your hard cheeses in an airtight container, you'll be able to enjoy them for several months.

Cheesy Spinach Bake

This golden puffed spinach casserole is made delicious by the addition of creamy, melty cheeses. This recipe is gluten-free.

Yield: 7 servings
Prep time: 5 minutes
Cook time: 1 hour
Serving size: ½ cup
Each serving has:
201 calories
12 g fat
7 g saturated fat
7 g carbohydrates
2 g fiber
17 g protein
462 mg sodium

2 large eggs, at room temperature

⅓ cup ground garbanzo and fava beans

1 (10-oz.) pkg. frozen chopped spinach, thawed

1½ cups low-fat, 1-percent-milk cottage cheese

1½ cups shredded cheddar cheese

⅛ tsp. fine sea salt

1. Preheat oven to 350°F.

2. In a large bowl, whisk eggs until lemon-colored. Whisk in ground beans. Add spinach, cottage cheese, cheddar cheese, and sea salt. Stir until blended.

3. Spoon mixture into a 1-quart baking dish coated with cooking spray. Bake, uncovered, for 1 hour or until the top is golden and puffy.

 For Good Measure

Moms can't always be right. Carrots are full of antioxidants and are good for you, but spinach is the vegetable to munch on for eye health.

Creamed Lima Beans

Tender, sweet beans are coated with a creamy white sauce. Enjoy its velvety texture without the taste of a raw flour thickener. This recipe is gluten-free.

3 cups fresh or frozen lima beans	**1⅛ cups Versatile Flourless White Sauce (recipe later in this chapter)**

1. Place lima beans in a medium saucepan. Cover with water by 1 inch. Bring to a boil over high heat. Skim foam, if necessary.

2. Reduce heat to low. Cover and simmer for 20 minutes or until tender. Drain.

3. Add Versatile Flourless White Sauce, and stir to coat evenly. Serve hot.

XXXX **No-Flour Power** _____

A basic white sauce can liven up any number of ho-hum veggies or make your favorites even more delicious. Stir it into asparagus, brussels sprouts, carrots, peas, mushrooms, and more.

Yield: 6 servings
Prep time: 2 minutes
Cook time: 30 minutes
Serving size: ½ cup
Each serving has:
93 calories
1 g fat
0 g saturated fat
16 g carbohydrates
4 g fiber
6 g protein
10 mg sodium

Cheddar Cheese Sauce

This smooth, creamy sauce enjoys a mild cheddar flavor with a speck of spice from cayenne. This recipe is gluten-free.

Yield: 10 servings
Prep time: 2 minutes
Cook time: 24 minutes
Serving size: ¼ cup
Each serving has:
100 calories
7 g fat
4 g saturated fat
6 g carbohydrates
0 g fiber
4 g protein
156 mg sodium

¼ cup unsalted butter

¼ cup stone-ground brown rice

¼ tsp. fine sea salt

2 TB. prepared yellow mustard

2 cups fat-free milk

⅛ tsp. cayenne pepper

½ cup shredded cheddar cheese

1. In a small saucepan over low heat, melt butter until bubbly (about 5 minutes). Whisk in stone-ground brown rice and sea salt. Whisk for 2 minutes or until bubbly.

2. Whisk in yellow mustard, milk, and cayenne pepper. Cook, whisking slowly, for 15 minutes or until thickened.

3. Whisk in cheese until melted and sauce is smooth. Serve hot over your favorite vegetables.

XXXX No-Flour Power

If your saucepan has a nonstick coating, you'll want to opt for a silicone or other nonscratching whisk, because a traditional stainless-steel whisk may harm your saucepan's finish.

Versatile Flourless White Sauce

Traditionally a butter-and-flour-thickened sauce, this seasoned cream sauce makes a tasty alternative. This recipe is gluten-free.

2 TB. unsalted butter

2 TB. stone-ground brown rice

Pinch fine sea salt

Pinch freshly ground black pepper

1 cup fat-free milk

Yield: 9 servings	
Prep time: 1 minute	
Cook time: 10 minutes	
Serving size: 2 tablespoons	
Each serving has:	
40 calories	
3 g fat	
2 g saturated fat	
3 g carbohydrates	
0 g fiber	
1 g protein	
45 mg sodium	

1. In a small saucepan, melt butter over medium-low heat until it starts to bubble.

2. Gradually whisk in stone-ground brown rice. Add sea salt and black pepper.

3. Gradually whisk in milk, whisking until smooth. Cook, whisking occasionally, for 5 minutes or until mixture bubbles and thickens. Remove from the heat.

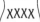

No-Flour Power

Stone-ground brown rice is a good flour substitute when you need a thickener.

Country Chicken Gravy

Pour this creamy, thick, chicken-broth-based gravy over your favorite chicken dishes, brown rice sides, sprouted-grain stuffing, and more. This recipe is gluten-free if the chicken is gluten-free.

Yield: 4 servings	
Prep time: 1 minute	
Cook time: 7 to 9 minutes	
Serving size: ¼ cup	

Each serving has:

76 calories

6 g fat

4 g saturated fat

5 g carbohydrates

0 g fiber

1 g protein

164 mg sodium

2 TB. unsalted butter

2 TB. stone-ground brown rice

⅛ tsp. fine sea salt

⅛ tsp. freshly ground black pepper

¾ cup fat-free, reduced-sodium chicken broth

¼ cup fat-free milk

1. Melt butter in a small saucepan over medium heat until bubbly. Whisk in stone-ground brown rice, sea salt, and black pepper until moistened.

2. Slowly whisk in chicken broth and milk until smooth. Continue whisking for 3 to 5 minutes or until thickened and bubbling. Serve hot.

For Good Measure

Peppercorns are available dried in both white and black options. If you don't care for black flecks in light sauces and gravies, opt for white peppercorns. White peppercorns are milder than their black counterparts so you may want to increase the amount to taste.

Casa-Style Spanish Rice

Tangy tomatoes and sautéed onions and green bell peppers brighten the nutlike flavor of more healthful brown rice seasoned with a blend of savory spices. This recipe is gluten-free.

2 tsp. extra-virgin olive oil

1 small yellow onion, diced

½ large green bell pepper, diced

2 medium cloves garlic, minced

2 cups cooked long-grain brown rice

1 tsp. chili powder

¼ tsp. ground cumin

¼ tsp. ground dried thyme

¼ tsp. fine sea salt

1 (14½-oz.) can petite-diced tomatoes, undrained

Yield: 7 servings
Prep time: 2 minutes
Cook time: 22 minutes
Serving size: ½ cup
Each serving has:
91 calories
2 g fat
0 g saturated fat
16 g carbohydrates
2 g fiber
2 g protein
194 mg sodium

1. Heat extra-virgin olive oil in a large skillet over medium heat. Sauté onion and green bell pepper for 5 minutes or until softened, stirring frequently. Reduce heat to medium-low. Stir in garlic. Sauté for 2 minutes or until garlic is golden.

2. Add brown rice, chili powder, cumin, thyme, and sea salt. Stir to combine. Cook for 5 minutes, stirring occasionally.

3. Stir in tomatoes. Cook for 10 minutes, stirring occasionally. Serve hot.

 For Good Measure

While brown rice does take longer to cook than white rice, you can easily keep cooked brown rice on hand to use as needed. Prepare brown rice when you have the time, and then freeze it in 1- or 2-cup portions. Thaw as needed.

Part 5

Dilemma-Solving Desserts

While eating three nutritious meals a day, you'll still want a sweet treat now and then. Everywhere you look, though, those scrumptious desserts are made with flours, starches, and sugars.

While unhealthful ingredients remain dessert perennials, a few substitutions and more healthful ingredients will have your sweet tooth smiling. Treat yourself to better-choice cakes, cookies, pies, puddings, and more end-of-meal delights.

Chapter 17

Best-Choice Cakes, Cookies, and More

In This Chapter

- ◆ Creamy cheesecake, chocolate cake, and cupcakes baked without flour
- ◆ Everyone's favorite cookies stirred up the flour-free way
- ◆ Chocolate lovers' treats of scrumptious brownies and truffles

Baked goods are notoriously full of flour. And while you may want to take a pass on the dessert tray, with our alternatives you can still delight in decadent treats without the accompanying guilt. Flour alternatives bake up into luscious desserts that'll satisfy your sweet tooth.

What's in Store

If you're preparing baked goods for an event—the school bake sale, a carry-in potluck, your dinner party tonight—storage is low on your list of concerns. However, if you're baking up treats for your family, there's a chance (albeit a slim chance) that you'll need to store your scrumptious creations beyond removal from the oven.

Certain baked goods must be refrigerated. Any desserts that include cream cheese, whipped cream, meringue, or custard are best kept chilled (such as a cheesecake, lemon meringue pie, and Boston cream pie). A recipe should state when a dessert needs to be stored in the refrigerator. However, any baked good can be kept in an airtight container in the refrigerator. If the dessert should be served at room temperature, simply remove it from the refrigerator 10 to 20 minutes before serving time.

Desserts that don't require refrigeration can be left out the day they're baked. (Of course, foods will dry out faster if left uncovered.) Cookies and cakes can then be transferred to an airtight container where they'll keep for several days at room temperature. Pies should be moved into the refrigerator.

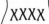

No-Flour Power

Even in an airtight container, the edges of a cut cake can dry out. To protect the cut surfaces, press pieces of wax paper onto the edges to keep them moist until serving time.

Creamy Crust-Free Cheesecake

This light and creamy cheesecake is topped with a sweet blueberry topping. This recipe is gluten-free.

3 (8-oz.) pkg. cream cheese, at room temperature

¾ cup plus 2 TB. agave nectar

¼ cup plus 2 tsp. ground almond meal

¼ tsp. fine sea salt

5 large eggs

1 cup fresh blueberries

Yield: 16 servings
Prep time: 20 minutes
Cook time: 50 to 60 minutes
Chill time: 8 hours
Serving size: 1 slice
Each serving has:
247 calories
17 g fat
10 g saturated fat
17 g carbohydrates
0 g fiber
6 g protein
182 mg sodium

1. Preheat oven to 325°F.

2. In a large bowl, stir cream cheese until smooth. Add ¾ cup agave nectar, and stir until blended thoroughly. Add ¼ cup ground almond meal and sea salt. Stir until blended. Add eggs, 1 at a time, stirring until blended thoroughly. (Blend with an electric mixer if preferred.)

3. Turn mixture into a 10-inch deep pie plate. Bake for 50 to 60 minutes or until top is set. (Center may appear wet; test for dryness by touching.) Let stand to cool slightly.

4. Meanwhile, combine blueberries and 2 tablespoons agave nectar in a small bowl. Using the back of a fork, coarsely mash blueberries until agave nectar is stained purple. Stir in 2 teaspoons ground almond meal until blended. Spread evenly over the top of cheesecake.

5. Cover and refrigerate overnight or until well chilled. Cut cheesecake into 16 slices to serve. Refrigerate leftovers.

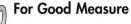 **For Good Measure**

Don't be concerned if the partially baked cheesecake is puffed up over the rim of the pie plate when you check on it through your oven's window. The cheesecake will settle when cooled, forming a rimmed "crust."

Golden Almond Cupcakes

Moist and tender, these sweet, slightly nutty treats can be enjoyed with or without frosting. This recipe is gluten-free.

Yield: 12 servings
Prep time: 15 minutes
Cook time: 20 minutes
Serving size: 1 cupcake
Each serving has:
197 calories
9 g fat
4 g saturated fat
25 g carbohydrates
5 g fiber
5 g protein
141 mg sodium

½ TB. fresh lemon juice

½ cup fat-free milk

½ cup ground almond meal

½ cup ground amaranth

½ cup ground coconut

1 tsp. baking soda

¾ tsp. xanthan gum

2 large eggs, at room temperature

⅔ cup agave nectar

¼ cup unsalted butter, melted

2 tsp. vanilla extract

Raspberry Cream Cheese Frosting (recipe later in this chapter), optional

1. Preheat oven to 350°F.

2. Pour lemon juice into milk. Set aside to curdle while you prepare the remaining ingredients.

3. In a medium bowl, combine ground almond meal, ground amaranth, ground coconut, baking soda, and xanthan gum. Stir to mix.

4. In a large bowl, whisk eggs until lemon-colored. Whisk in agave nectar until well blended. Whisk in melted butter and vanilla extract until blended. Stir in dry ingredients until moistened. Stir in curdled milk until blended. (Batter will be thick.)

5. Spoon batter into muffin cups lined with paper baking cups, filling ¾ full. Bake for 20 minutes or until a cake tester or a wooden toothpick inserted in the center comes out clean. Cool completely on a wire rack before removing from the pan. Frost with Raspberry Cream Cheese Frosting, if desired. Cover and refrigerate if frosted.

For Good Measure

Pure vanilla extract is more costly than the imitation extracts available because vanilla beans are hand-picked and hand-prepared. Still, little is called for in any recipe, and the superior flavor is worth the price.

Creamy Chocolate Cake

Moist, dense, lightly chocolate-flavored, this two-layer cake tastes sweet and yummy. This recipe is gluten-free.

1 TB. fresh lemon juice	2 large eggs, at room temperature
1 cup fat-free milk	1 small ripe banana, mashed
1 cup ground amaranth	½ cup agave nectar
1 cup ground coconut	1½ oz. unsweetened chocolate, melted
1 tsp. xanthan gum	1 tsp. vanilla extract
1 tsp. baking soda	Raspberry Cream Cheese Frosting (recipe later in this chapter), optional
½ tsp. fine sea salt	
½ cup unsalted butter, at room temperature	
¾ cup date sugar	

Yield: 16 servings
Prep time: 25 minutes
Cook time: 25 minutes
Serving size: 1 slice
Each serving has:
242 calories
10 g fat
7 g saturated fat
32 g carbohydrates
7 g fiber
5 g protein
194 mg sodium

1. Preheat oven to 350°F.

2. Pour lemon juice into milk. Set aside to curdle while you prepare the remaining ingredients.

3. In a medium bowl, combine ground amaranth, ground coconut, xanthan gum, baking soda, and sea salt. Stir to mix.

4. In a large mixing bowl, combine butter and date sugar. Beat with an electric mixer on medium-low speed for 4 to 5 minutes or until blended. Add eggs, 1 at a time, mixing until blended. Add banana, agave nectar, chocolate, and vanilla extract. Mix until blended.

5. Alternately, add dry ingredients and curdled milk, beginning and ending with dry ingredients. Mix until blended. (Batter will be thick.)

6. Coat 2 (9-inch) layer pans with cooking spray. Evenly divide batter between pans and smooth tops. Bake for 25 minutes or until a cake tester or a wooden toothpick inserted into the center comes out clean. Cool completely on a wire rack before frosting, as desired.

7. If frosting with Raspberry Cream Cheese Frosting, spread ½ cup frosting over one layer. Place second layer over top upside down. Spread remaining frosting over top. Cover and refrigerate.

No-Flour Power

Chocolate can be melted in the top of a double boiler over simmering water, in a heavy saucepan over low heat, or in the microwave in short intervals on 50 percent power. Stir the chocolate frequently to check its status, as it will be melted before it appears to be melted.

Raspberry Cream Cheese Frosting

This lavender-tinged frosting offers the flavor of cream cheese sweetened with luscious red raspberries. This recipe is gluten-free.

Yield: 12 servings
Prep time: 10 minutes
Serving size: 1½ table-spoons
Each serving has:
63 calories
3 g fat
2 g saturated fat
7 g carbohydrates
0 g fiber
1 g protein
57 mg sodium

6 oz. Neufchâtel cheese, at room temperature

3 TB. all-fruit seedless, red raspberry spreadable fruit

3 TB. agave nectar

1. In a medium bowl, cut Neufchâtel cheese into small pieces. Add spreadable fruit, and stir until smooth.

2. Add agave nectar. Stir until smooth. Frost cake or cupcakes as desired. Cover and chill until serving time. Refrigerate any leftovers.

Variation: Substitute your favorite smooth fruit spread in the same quantity.

For Good Measure

The Neufchâtel cheese called for in this cookbook isn't the soft yellow French cheese, but the low-fat cream cheese labeled as Neufchâtel cheese. Look for it in your supermarket's refrigerated case next to the regular and fat-free blocks of cream cheese.

Tempting Pecan Tassies

The tender, golden crust holds meaty pecans in a sweet syrup for a bite-size taste of pecan pie. This recipe is gluten-free.

1 (8-oz.) pkg. Neufchâtel cheese or low-fat cream cheese

½ cup unsalted butter, softened

2½ cups ground almond meal

1 large egg, at room temperature

½ cup honey

1 TB. unsalted butter, melted

1 tsp. vanilla extract

1½ cups chopped pecans

Yield: 32 servings
Prep time: 25 minutes
Chill time: 2 hours
Cook time: 20 minutes
Serving size: 1 cookie
Each serving has:
160 calories
13 g fat
4 g saturated fat
7 g carbohydrates
1 g fiber
3 g protein
31 mg sodium

1. In a medium bowl, combine Neufchâtel cheese and softened butter. Stir until thoroughly blended. Add ground almond meal a little at a time, stirring until well blended. Cover and chill for at least 2 hours or until dough is very firm.

2. Preheat oven to 350°F.

3. In another medium bowl, whisk egg until lemon-colored. Whisk in honey until blended. Stir in melted butter and vanilla extract. Stir in pecans to coat evenly.

4. Working quickly, shape dough into 1-inch balls and place in the cups of nonstick mini muffin pans. Using a mini-tart shaper, the back of a small scoop, or another rounded spoon, press each ball so that it covers the inside of the mini muffin cups.

5. Fill cups with pecan mixture, continually stirring pecan mixture before filling cups to keep pecans evenly coated. (Do not overfill cups.) Bake for 20 minutes or until cups are golden-brown.

6. Cool completely in the mini muffin pans on a wire rack. Let stand for at least 2 hours after cooling before removing from the cups. (The dough is delicate, and the longer the cookies stand, the easier they are to remove from the cups.) Refrigerate any leftovers, bringing back to room temperature before serving.

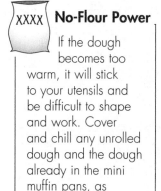

No-Flour Power

If the dough becomes too warm, it will stick to your utensils and be difficult to shape and work. Cover and chill any unrolled dough and the dough already in the mini muffin pans, as needed.

Steel-Cut Oatmeal and Raisin Cookies

These thick, chewy cookies enjoy a hearty oat flavor sweetened by bits of raisins and cinnamon.

Yield: 30 servings
Prep time: 30 minutes
Cook time: 15 minutes per batch
Serving size: 1 cookie
Each serving has:
71 calories
4 g fat
2 g saturated fat
8 g carbohydrates
1 g fiber
1 g protein
32 mg sodium

2 cups cooked steel-cut oats, hot

½ cup raisins

½ cup unsalted butter, melted

½ cup date sugar

1 large egg, at room temperature

½ tsp. vanilla extract

½ cup ground quinoa

¼ tsp. xanthan gum

¼ tsp. baking soda

¼ tsp. fine sea salt

½ tsp. ground cinnamon

1. In a medium bowl, combine hot, cooked steel-cut oats and raisins. Stir. Set aside to cool.

2. Meanwhile, preheat oven to 350°F.

3. In a large bowl, combine butter, date sugar, egg, and vanilla extract. Stir until well blended.

4. In a small bowl, combine ground quinoa, xanthan gum, baking soda, sea salt, and cinnamon. Stir to mix. Add to butter mixture, and stir until moistened. Add steel-cut oats mixture, and stir until blended.

5. Using a 1-tablespoon cookie scoop, drop dough by rounded scoops onto ungreased cookie sheets 2 inches apart. Bake for 15 minutes or until browned. Remove to a wire rack to cool.

For Good Measure

Seedless Thompson grapes are used to make both dark and golden raisins. Dark raisins are sun-dried; golden raisins are dried in a dehydrator and preserved with sulfur dioxide.

Natural Peanut Butter Cookies

The taste of peanut butter pure and simple can be enjoyed, unadulterated by flour, in these cookies. This recipe is gluten-free if the peanut butter is gluten-free.

1 cup natural salt-free peanut butter

1 cup date sugar

2 large eggs, at room temperature

1. Preheat oven to 350°F.

2. In a large bowl, combine peanut butter, date sugar, and eggs. Stir until well blended.

3. Using a 1-tablespoon cookie scoop or tablespoon, drop dough 2 inches apart onto ungreased cookie sheets. Using the tines of a large fork, gently press a criss-cross pattern into each dough ball, flattening slightly.

4. Bake for 6 to 8 minutes or until browned. Cool on the cookie sheet for 1 minute. Carefully remove cookies to a wire rack to cool completely.

Yield: 24 servings
Prep time: 10 minutes
Cook time: 6 to 8 minutes per batch
Serving size: 1 cookie
Each serving has:
102 calories
6 g fat
1 g saturated fat
8 g carbohydrates
1 g fiber
4 g protein
5 mg sodium

For Good Measure

Fresh dates are available in three types: soft, semidry, and dry. Date sugar is simply ground dried dates, and therefore contains the fiber, vitamins, and minerals found in the fruit.

Chocolate-Walnut Brownies

These nut-studded, cake-style brownies conquer your chocolate craving. This recipe is gluten-free.

Yield: 16 servings
Prep time: 15 minutes
Cook time: 29 to 34 minutes
Serving size: 1 brownie
Each serving has:
175 calories
11 g fat
5 g saturated fat
17 g carbohydrates
3 g fiber
3 g protein
72 mg sodium

5 TB. unsalted butter, cut in pieces	¼ tsp. fine sea salt
2 oz. unsweetened chocolate	¾ cup chopped walnuts
½ cup ground amaranth	2 large eggs, at room temperature
¼ cup ground coconut	½ cup agave nectar
¼ cup ground sorghum	½ tsp. vanilla extract
¼ tsp. baking soda	

1. Preheat oven to 350°F.

2. In a small saucepan over low heat, melt butter and chocolate, stirring occasionally (about 4 minutes). Remove from heat and cool.

3. In a medium bowl, combine ground amaranth, ground coconut, ground sorghum, baking soda, and sea salt. Stir to mix. Stir in walnuts to coat.

4. In a large bowl, whisk eggs until lemon-colored. Whisk in agave nectar and vanilla extract. Stir in chocolate mixture until blended. Add dry ingredients, and stir until moistened.

5. Coat an 8×8×2 baking pan with cooking spray. Pour batter into pan and smooth top. Bake for 25 to 30 minutes or until a cake tester or a wooden toothpick inserted in the center comes out clean. Cool completely on a wire rack. Cut into 2-inch squares to serve.

XXXX **No-Flour Power**

If you're baking in dark-finished baking pans or glass-type baking dishes, reduce the oven temperature by 25°F to avoid overcooking.

Almond-Dusted Chocolate Truffles

Savor a sweet, creamy bite of chocolate in these truffles with a bit of almond flavor and crunch. This recipe is gluten-free.

1 cup date sugar	**4 oz. Neufchâtel cheese**
½ cup natural unsweetened cocoa powder	**½ tsp. almond extract**
	2 TB. ground almond meal

Yield: 12 servings
Prep time: 15 minutes
Chill time: 2 hours
Serving size: 2 truffles
Each serving has:
92 calories
3 g fat
1 g saturated fat
14 g carbohydrates
1 g fiber
2 g protein
38 mg sodium

1. In a food processor, combine date sugar, cocoa powder, Neufchâtel cheese, and almond extract. Process on high speed for 30 seconds or until dough forms a ball.

2. Roll dough into 1-inch balls. Roll in ground almond meal measured onto wax paper. Coat evenly, pressing gently into surface of truffles. Cover and chill in a single layer for at least 2 hours before serving. Refrigerate leftovers.

For Good Measure

Date sugar, because it's simply ground dried dates and not really a sugar such as those processed from cane and beets, does not "melt" into your recipes.

Chapter 18

Revised Pies and Other Happy Endings

In This Chapter

- ◆ Flour-free pie crust packed with healthful fillings
- ◆ Fruity crisp and cobbler for easy dessert treats
- ◆ Creamy puddings and frosty yogurt for lip-smacking spoonfuls

You can create desserts that will not only satisfy your sweet tooth but also provide the perfect ending to a great meal. You'll be able to enjoy many of your traditional favorites—only flour-free.

Only Fools Rush In

As discussed in earlier chapters, the goal is to stabilize your blood glucose level and, in doing so, avoid an increase in insulin. This increase in blood glucose is often due to the consumption of sugar-laden, end-of-meal treats. A successful day of healthful eating can easily be sabotaged by one detrimental dessert. The recipes that follow will help you overcome this pitfall without having to deprive yourself of the foods you enjoy.

For this reason, none of the recipes in this chapter (or in this cookbook) contain any refined sugars. Instead, your taste buds will be dazzled and your sweet cravings satisfied by eating desserts made with natural alternatives. We've employed more healthful sugar substitutes, such as stevia, agave nectar, honey, concentrated fruit juices, and date sugar. You might also like to try maple syrup, sweet fiber, barley malt, and more natural choices to sweeten things up.

For Good Measure

Honey is a natural sweetener made by bees using the nectars of flowers. Because it provides a similar level of sweetness, it's an excellent substitute for sugar. This more healthful alternative contains trace amounts of many essential vitamins and minerals. Recent research now suggests that honey may also benefit our immune system as an antibacterial and antioxidant.

Buttery Almond Pie Crust

Delicate and flaky, this pie crust offers a mild, unobtrusive flavor with just a hint of nutty taste. This recipe is gluten-free.

¾ **cup ground quinoa**

½ **cup ground almond meal**

½ **tsp. xanthan gum**

6 TB. **unsalted butter, at room temperature**

3 to 4 TB. **cold water, or as needed**

Yield: 8 servings	
Prep time: 20 minutes	
Cook time: 20 minutes (optional)	
Serving size: 1 slice	
Each serving has:	
164 calories	
13 g fat	
6 g saturated fat	
10 g carbohydrates	
1 g fiber	
3 g protein	
4 mg sodium	

1. In a medium bowl, combine ground quinoa, ground almond meal, and xanthan gum. Stir to mix.

2. Cut butter into small pieces. Using a pastry blender or two butter knives, cut butter into dry ingredients until crumbly. Add cold water, 1 tablespoon at a time, stirring into mixture with a fork. Add just enough water to make a dough that forms a ball and cleans the side of the bowl.

3. Turn out dough onto a work surface lightly dusted with additional ground quinoa. Flatten dough with the heels of your hands that are dusted with ground quinoa and flip. Redust the work surface as necessary. With a dusted rolling pin, roll out dough to an 11-inch circle.

4. To transfer dough to a 9-inch pie plate, gently fold dough in half and then in quarters. Place the point of dough in the center of the pie plate. Carefully unfold dough, and press into the pie plate. Pinch dough around the edge to crimp the crust. Prick all over with the tines of a fork.

5. Chill dough while you prepare a pie filling, and bake according to the pie recipe directions. Or, to pre-bake crust, bake in a preheated 350°F oven for 20 minutes or until browned. Cool completely on a wire rack before filling.

 For Good Measure

Traditional pastries perform best with the least amount of handling possible. But don't be afraid to reroll this pie crust if necessary—practice will provide the delicate touch needed to work with this dough. If you experience only a small break, the dough can be repaired right in the pie pan.

Sweet Strawberry Pie

Luscious summer berries pack this delicate buttery pie crust. This recipe is gluten-free.

Yield: 8 servings
Prep time: 25 minutes
Cook time: 3 to 5 minutes
Chill time: 1 hour
Serving size: 1 slice
Each serving has:
247 calories
13 g fat
6 g saturated fat
26 g carbohydrates
3 g fiber
6 g protein
6 mg sodium

24 packets stevia (equal to 1 cup sugar)

2 TB. stone-ground brown rice

1 cup boiling water

½ oz. (2 envelopes) unflavored gelatin

6 drops red food coloring, or as desired

1½ lb. fresh strawberries, hulled

1 (9-inch) prepared and baked Buttery Almond Pie Crust (recipe earlier in this chapter)

1. In a small saucepan, combine stevia and stone-ground brown rice. Stir to mix. Gradually pour in boiling water while stirring. Cook over medium heat, stirring constantly, for 3 to 5 minutes or until mixture begins to thicken and bubble.

2. Turn off the heat. Very slowly stir in gelatin, stirring until smooth. Stir in food coloring until evenly colored. Set aside to cool for about 15 minutes until cooled but not set.

3. Meanwhile, arrange strawberries points up in prepared pre-baked Buttery Almond Pie Crust, tipping berries back against the outer edge of crust. Pour cooled gelatin mixture between strawberries evenly across pie.

4. Cover and chill for at least 1 hour or until gelatin is set. Cut into 8 slices to serve. Refrigerate any leftovers.

No-Flour Power _____

Unflavored gelatin is a single-ingredient product that provides gelling properties without the starches, sugars, and additives that show up on ingredients lists of flavored gelatins.

Presentation Pumpkin Pie

The buttery almond crust doesn't distract from the mildly spiced pure pumpkin flavor filling this pie. This recipe is gluten-free.

2 large eggs, at room temperature

1 (15-ounce) can pure pumpkin

½ cup fat-free plain yogurt

⅓ cup agave nectar

1 tsp. pumpkin pie spice

1 (9-inch) prepared Buttery Almond Pie Crust (recipe earlier in this chapter)

Yield: 8 servings
Prep time: 10 minutes
Cook time: 70 to 80 minutes
Serving size: 1 slice
Each serving has:
255 calories
14 g fat
6 g saturated fat
26 g carbohydrates
2 g fiber
6 g protein
35 mg sodium

1. Preheat the oven to 400°F.

2. In a medium bowl, whisk eggs vigorously for 3 minutes or until thickened and frothy. Add pumpkin, yogurt, agave nectar, and pumpkin pie spice. Stir until well blended. Spoon into Buttery Almond Pie Crust, and smooth top.

3. Bake for 10 minutes. Reduce oven temperature to 350°F. Continue baking for 60 to 70 minutes or until filling is set and a knife inserted into the center leaves a slit. During baking, once the crust is browned, protect it with a pie shield or cover the edge with aluminum foil to prevent burning. Cool completely on a wire rack before cutting. Sprinkle a pinch of pumpkin pie spice over the top of the pie, if desired.

4. To serve, cut into 8 slices. Serve warm or cold. Refrigerate any leftovers.

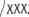 **No-Flour Power** _____

You'll find cans of pumpkin and cans of pumpkin pie filling side by side in your supermarket's baking aisle. Pumpkin pie filling is already spiced and sweetened. Choose the can that boasts pure pumpkin.

Peach Almond Crisp

These sweet, spiced peaches are topped with a crisp and crunchy double-almond crumble. This recipe is gluten-free.

Yield: 7 servings
Prep time: 12 minutes
Cook time: 25 minutes
Serving size: ½ cup
Each serving has:
276 calories
14 g fat
5 g saturated fat
33 g carbohydrates
3 g fiber
4 g protein
1 mg sodium

3½ cups peeled, sliced peaches

1 TB. fresh lemon juice

¼ cup honey

¼ tsp. almond extract

¼ tsp. ground cinnamon

¼ tsp. ground nutmeg

¾ cup ground almond meal

½ cup date sugar

¼ cup unsalted butter, at room temperature

¼ cup sliced almonds

1. Preheat oven to 350°F.

2. In a medium bowl, combine peaches and lemon juice. Stir to coat. Add honey, almond extract, cinnamon, and nutmeg. Stir to coat evenly. Spoon into an 8×8×2 baking dish coated with cooking spray.

3. In another medium bowl, combine ground almond meal and date sugar. Stir. Cut butter into small pieces. Using a pastry blender or two butter knives, cut butter into dry ingredients until crumbly. Add sliced almonds. Stir into crumbs, breaking almonds into pieces as you incorporate them. Evenly crumble almond mixture over top of peach mixture in the baking dish.

4. Bake, uncovered, for 25 minutes or until bubbly and topping is crisped and golden brown. Serve hot with sugar-free ice cream, if desired. Refrigerate any leftovers.

> **XXXX** **No-Flour Power**
>
> To peel a peach easily, cut an X in the blossom end with a sharp knife. Submerge the peach in boiling water for 20 seconds. Remove and, using the tip of the knife, loosen the peel from the intersection of the X. The skin should easily peel away.

Bubbly Blueberry Cobbler

Bursting with sweet blueberry flavor, this cobbler is capped off with a delicate almond-flavored crust. This recipe is gluten-free.

2 tsp. plus 1 TB. fresh lemon juice

⅓ cup fat-free milk

1 TB. stone-ground brown rice

3½ cups fresh blueberries

5 TB. unsalted butter, cut into small pieces

¼ cup plus ½ TB. agave nectar

¼ tsp. ground nutmeg

1 cup ground almond meal

½ TB. baking soda

½ tsp. ground cinnamon

¼ tsp. fine sea salt

Yield: 7 servings
Prep time: 23 minutes
Cook time: 30 minutes
Serving size: ½ cup
Each serving has:
267 calories
16 g fat
6 g saturated fat
26 g carbohydrates
4 g fiber
5 g protein
361 mg sodium

1. Preheat oven to 350°F.

2. Pour 2 teaspoons lemon juice into milk. Set aside to curdle.

3. In a small bowl, pour 1 tablespoon lemon juice into stone-ground brown rice. Stir into a paste. Set aside.

4. In a medium bowl, combine blueberries, 2 tablespoons butter, ¼ cup agave nectar, and nutmeg. Stir in stone-ground brown rice paste until blended. Spoon mixture into an 8×8×2 baking dish coated with cooking spray.

5. In another medium bowl, combine ground almond meal, baking soda, cinnamon, and sea salt. Stir to mix. Using a pastry blender or two butter knives, cut in 3 tablespoons butter until crumbly. Stir in ½ tablespoon agave nectar and curdled milk until blended. Spoon over filling.

6. Bake, uncovered, for 30 minutes or until bubbly and topping is browned. Let stand for at least 15 minutes before serving. Serve warm or cold with sugar-free ice cream, if desired. Refrigerate any leftovers.

> XXXX **No-Flour Power**
>
> Store spices in a cool, dark place to ensure the best quality. You shouldn't keep your spice collection above the stove or in the cabinet next to the oven. The steam and heat cause temperature fluctuations, deteriorating the flavor and increasing the possibility of caking.

Mixed Berries Frosty Yogurt

This frozen treat combines the flavors of all your favorite summer berries any time of the year. This recipe is gluten-free.

Yield: 8 servings
Prep time: 2 minutes
Chill time: 2 hours
Serving size: ½ cup
Each serving has:
65 calories
0 g fat
0 g saturated fat
13 g carbohydrates
2 g fiber
3 g protein
35 mg sodium

1 (15-ounce) pkg. unsweetened, frozen mixed berries

1½ cups fat-free plain yogurt

½ cup fresh orange juice

1 TB. agave nectar

1. In a blender, combine frozen mixed berries, yogurt, orange juice, and agave nectar. Cover and blend on high speed or the ice-crush option for 30 seconds or until blended. Stop to scrape down sides as needed.

2. Pour mixture into an 8×2 round dish or other shallow dish. Cover and freeze for at least 2 hours or until icy (about the consistency of sorbet). Serve immediately upon scooping into dessert dishes or serving bowls. Store any leftovers in the freezer.

Variation: Double the agave nectar if you prefer this frosty yogurt sweeter. Substitute a 15-ounce package of any unsweetened frozen fruit.

No-Flour Power

XXXX

You'll need 2 to 3 medium navel oranges to render ½ cup fresh juice.

Banana-Nana Pudding

Over-the-top bananas! A bowl of this pudding offers the extra sweetness of mashed ripe bananas, as well as the texture of sliced bananas. This recipe is gluten-free.

⅓ cup ground garbanzo and fava beans

¼ tsp. fine sea salt

3 large eggs, at room temperature

⅓ cup agave nectar

3 medium very ripe bananas

2 cups fat-free milk

½ tsp. vanilla extract

2 TB. unsalted butter, at room temperature

2 medium yellow bananas, thinly sliced

Yield: 12 servings
Prep time: 15 minutes
Cook time: 50 minutes
Serving size: ½ cup
Each serving has:
130 calories
4 g fat
2 g saturated fat
20 g carbohydrates
2 g fiber
4 g protein
85 mg sodium

1. In a large saucepan, combine ground beans and sea salt. Stir.

2. In a small bowl, whisk eggs until lemon-colored. Whisk in agave nectar until well blended.

3. In another small bowl, mash ripe bananas with a fork until well puréed.

4. Whisk egg mixture into dry ingredients in the saucepan. Whisk in puréed bananas. With the saucepan over low heat, whisk in milk. Whisk slowly for 50 minutes or until thickened to the point when the mixture is displaced by whisking.

5. Remove the saucepan from the heat. Continue to whisk slowly for 5 minutes or until mixture is slightly cooled. Whisk in vanilla extract and butter until blended.

6. Spoon pudding into a serving dish. Stir in sliced bananas. Cover and chill for at least 2 hours or until cold before serving.

Variation: If not serving immediately, chill without stirring in the sliced bananas to prevent browning. Just before serving, stir the sliced bananas into the cold pudding.

 For Good Measure

When your bananas start to turn brown, their starches convert to sugars, making them mushy, sweeter, and perfect for mashing into baked goods and desserts.

Creamy Chocolate Pudding

Thick, creamy, chocolaty spoonfuls of this pudding will bring a smile to your lips. This recipe is gluten-free.

Yield: 4 servings
Prep time: 5 minutes
Cook time: 10 minutes
Chill time: 8 hours
Serving size: ½ cup
Each serving has:
163 calories
1 g fat
0 g saturated fat
33 g carbohydrates
3 g fiber
5 g protein
134 mg sodium

¼ **cup natural unsweetened cocoa powder**

¼ **cup stone-ground brown rice**

⅛ **tsp. fine sea salt**

2 **cups fat-free milk**

¼ **cup agave nectar**

1 **tsp. vanilla extract**

1. In a medium saucepan, combine cocoa powder, stone-ground brown rice, and sea salt. Stir to mix.

2. Place the saucepan over medium heat and gradually add milk, whisking to blend. Gradually whisk in agave nectar. Continue to cook, whisking constantly, until mixture begins to simmer.

3. For 2 minutes, whisk vigorously while mixture simmers and boils. Scrape the bottom of the saucepan to keep milk from scorching.

4. Remove from the heat, and continue whisking for 1 minute to cool slightly. Whisk in vanilla extract until blended. Transfer pudding to a small bowl. Cover and chill overnight or until cold and set.

No-Flour Power

If you don't care for the skin that forms on the top of set pudding, it's easy to prevent by covering the pudding directly. Cut a piece of plastic wrap about twice as long as the bowl's width. Set the plastic wrap directly on the surface of the pudding, and then up the side of the bowl to seal off the surface.

Chocolate-Glazed Baked Pears

Sweet, tender pears, plated whole with stems intact and set off with a drizzle of subtle chocolate sauce, make a pretty presentation dessert or an easy everyday meal ending. This recipe is gluten-free.

6 ripe Bosc pears

1 TB. fresh lemon juice

2 TB. stone-ground brown rice

2 TB. fat-free milk

½ TB. natural unsweetened cocoa powder

2 TB. agave nectar

⅛ tsp. vanilla extract

Yield: 6 servings
Prep time: 20 minutes
Cook time: 1 hour
Serving size: 1 pear with 2 teaspoons chocolate glaze
Each serving has:
155 calories
1 g fat
0 g saturated fat
36 g carbohydrates
5 g fiber
1 g protein
3 mg sodium

1. Preheat the oven to 350°F.

2. Cut a thin slice from the bottom of each pear to allow it to stand upright. Peel pears. Using an apple corer or a melon baller, remove the bottom half of each core; leave the stem intact.

3. Arrange pears in a shallow baking dish or a pie plate. Spoon lemon juice over pears to coat evenly. Loosely cover pears with foil, cutting holes in the foil to place the stems through. Bake for 1 hour or until tender.

4. Meanwhile, whisk stone-ground brown rice into milk in a small bowl. Whisk in cocoa powder until smooth. Add agave nectar and vanilla extract. Stir to blend well.

5. Arrange baked pears on serving plates. To serve hot, drizzle chocolate glaze onto plates and over pears. To serve cold, cover and chill pears and chocolate glaze for at least 2 hours or until cold. Stir chocolate glaze to reblend and drizzle over the plates and chilled pears.

XXXX **No-Flour Power** _____

Pears are available for sale while still hard and not ripe. Store them at room temperature until the blossom ends soften slightly. Typically, pears will ripen in a couple days at room temperature. Keep an eye on them, as pears are quick to pass into grainy over-ripeness.

Glossary

adipose tissue   A type of connective tissue that stores cellular fat. The most common types in humans are subcutaneous and visceral fat. Subcutaneous is the type beneath the skin, while visceral is the type that surrounds internal organs. An elevated amount of visceral fat is linked to an increased risk of heart disease.

agave nectar   A natural sweetener derived from the agave plant grown in Mexico. Also, agave syrup.

al dente   Italian for "against the teeth." Refers to pasta or rice that's neither soft nor hard, but just slightly firm to the bite.

almonds   Mild, sweet, and crunchy nuts that combine nicely with creamy and sweet food items.

au gratin   The quick broiling of a dish before serving to brown the top ingredients. When used in a recipe name, the term often implies cheese and a creamy sauce.

bake   To cook in a dry oven. Dry-heat cooking often results in a crisping of the exterior of the food being cooked. Moist-heat cooking, through methods such as steaming, poaching, etc., brings a much different, moist quality to the food.

bamboo shoots   Crunchy, tasty white parts of the growing bamboo plant, often purchased canned.

barbecue   To cook something (usually meat) slowly over low heat, using charcoal and/or wood as a fuel source.

basil   A flavorful, almost sweet, resinous herb used in a variety of Italian and Mediterranean-style dishes. Often paired with tomatoes.

beat   To quickly mix ingredients.

Belgian endive   A plant that resembles a small, elongated, tightly packed head of romaine lettuce. The thick, crunchy, slightly bitter leaves can be broken off and used with dips and spreads.

black pepper   A biting and pungent seasoning, freshly ground pepper is a must for many dishes and adds an extra level of flavor.

blend   To completely mix something, usually with a blender or food processor, more slowly than beating.

blue cheese   A blue-veined cheese that crumbles easily and has a somewhat soft texture and strong taste, usually sold in a block. The color is from a flavorful, edible mold that is often added or injected into the cheese.

boil   To heat a liquid to a point where water is forced to turn into steam, causing the liquid to bubble. To boil something is to insert it into boiling water. A rapid boil is when a lot of bubbles form on the surface of the liquid.

breadcrumbs   Tiny pieces of crumbled dry bread, often used for a topping or coating.

broil   To cook in a dry oven beneath an overhead high-heat element.

broth   *See* stock.

brown   To cook in a skillet, turning, until the food's surface is seared and brown in color, adding richer, deeper flavor to the food.

brown rice   Whole-grain rice including the germ with a characteristic pale brown or tan color; more nutritious and flavorful than white rice.

calorie   The amount of energy required to raise the temperature of 1 gram of water 1 degree Celsius. This basic unit of energy is often called the small calorie. One-thousand small calories are known as a kilocalorie. A kilocalorie is the amount of energy contained in food and released upon digestion by the human body. Nutritional labels list kilocalories as "Calories."

capers   Flavorful buds of a Mediterranean plant, ranging in size from *nonpareil* (about the size of a small pea) to larger, grape-size caper berries produced in Spain. Available in brine or packed in salt.

caraway   A distinctive spicy seed used for bread, pork, cheese, and cabbage dishes. It is known to reduce stomach upset, which is why it is often paired with sauerkraut, for example.

carbohydrate   A nutritional component found in starches, sugars, fruits, and vegetables that causes a rise in blood glucose levels. Carbohydrates supply energy and many important nutrients, including vitamins, minerals, and antioxidants.

cayenne   A fiery spice made from ground chili peppers, especially the cayenne chili, a slender, red, and very hot pepper.

cheddar   The ubiquitous hard cow's milk cheese with a rich, buttery flavor that ranges from mellow to sharp. Originally produced in England, cheddar is now produced worldwide.

chili powder   A seasoning blend that includes chili pepper, cumin, garlic, and oregano. Proportions vary among different versions, but they all offer a warm, rich flavor.

chilis (or **chiles**)   Any one of many different "hot" peppers, ranging in intensity from the relatively mild ancho pepper to the blisteringly hot habañero.

chives   A member of the onion family, chives grow in bunches of long leaves that resemble tall grass or the green tops of onions and offer a light onion flavor.

cholesterol   A form of fat called a sterol found in animal and plant tissue. In humans, the liver manufactures cholesterol, and it's absorbed from food in the intestine. Cholesterol is a major component of blood plasma and cell membranes and is important for brain and nerve function. It is also a precursor in the production of vitamin D2, estrogen, testosterone, and cortisol.

chop   To cut into pieces, usually qualified by an adverb such as "*coarsely* chopped," or by a size measurement such as "chopped into ½-inch pieces." "Finely chopped" is much closer to minced.

cider vinegar   Vinegar produced from apple cider, popular in North America.

cilantro   A member of the parsley family and used in Mexican cooking (especially salsa) and some Asian dishes. Should be used in moderation, as the flavor can overwhelm. The seed of the cilantro plant is the spice coriander.

cinnamon A sweet, rich, aromatic spice commonly used in baking or desserts. Cinnamon can also be used for delicious and interesting entrées.

count In terms of seafood or other foods that come in small sizes, the number of that item that compose 1 pound. For example, 31 to 40 count shrimp are large appetizer shrimp often served with cocktail sauce; 51 to 60 count shrimp are much smaller.

croutons Cubes of bread, usually between ¼ and ½ inch in size—sometimes seasoned and baked, broiled, or fried to a crisp texture and used to garnish soups and salads.

cumin An earthy, smoky-tasting spice popular in Middle Eastern and Indian dishes. Cumin is a seed; ground cumin seed is the most common form used in cooking.

curd A gelatinous substance resulting from coagulated milk used to make cheese. Curd also refers to dishes of similar texture, such as dishes made with egg (lemon curd).

devein The removal of the dark vein from the back of a shrimp with a sharp knife.

dice To cut into small cubes about ¼-inch square.

Dijon mustard Hearty, spicy mustard made in the style of the Dijon region of France.

dill An herb perfect for eggs, salmon, cheese dishes, and vegetables (such as pickles!).

dollop A spoonful of something creamy and thick, such as sour cream or whipped cream.

double boiler A set of two pots designed to nest together, one inside the other, that provide consistent, moist heat for foods that need delicate treatment. The bottom pot holds water (not quite touching the bottom of the top pot); the top pot holds the ingredient you want to heat.

dredge To coat a piece of food with a dry substance such as flour or cornmeal.

drizzle To lightly sprinkle drops of a liquid over food, often as the finishing touch to a dish.

entrée The main dish in a meal. In France, however, the entrée is considered the first course.

essential amino acids Protein builders not produced by the body that need to be supplied in the daily diet.

extra-virgin olive oil   *See* olive oil.

feta   A white, crumbly, sharp, and salty cheese popular in Greek cooking and on salads. Traditional feta is usually made with sheep milk, but feta-style cheese can also be made from cow or goat milk.

fillet   A piece of meat or seafood with the bones removed.

flake   To break into thin sections, as with fish.

floret   The flower or bud end of broccoli or cauliflower.

fold   To combine a dense mixture with a light mixture by stirring with a circular action from the bottom of the bowl.

frittata   A skillet-cooked mixture of eggs and other ingredients that is not stirred but is cooked slowly and then either flipped or finished under the broiler.

fructose   Sugar naturally found in fruit, which is slightly sweeter than table sugar.

fry   To cook in a pan or on a griddle over direct heat, usually in hot fat or oil.

garbanzo beans (or **chickpeas**)   A yellow-gold, roundish bean used as the base ingredient in hummus. Chickpeas are high in fiber and low in fat.

garlic   A cousin of the onion, garlic is a pungent and flavorful element in many savory dishes. A garlic bulb contains multiple cloves. Each clove, when chopped, provides about 1 teaspoon garlic. Most recipes call for cloves or chopped garlic by the teaspoon.

garnish   An embellishment to a dish that enhances visual appeal, flavor, and/or texture.

ginger   Available in fresh root or dried, ground form, ginger adds a pungent, sweet, and spicy quality to a dish.

glucose   The simplest natural sugar.

grate   To shave into tiny pieces using a sharp rasp or grater.

grind   To reduce a large, hard substance, often a seasoning such as peppercorns, to the consistency of sand.

groat   The term for a cereal grain such as oats, wheat, or buckwheat that only has the outer shell or coating removed.

ground coconut   A low-carbohydrate flour substitute that contains the mineral manganese.

Gruyère   A rich, sharp cow milk cheese made in Switzerland that has a nutty flavor.

handful   An unscientific measurement; the amount of an ingredient you can hold in your hand.

hazelnuts (also **filberts**)   A sweet nut popular in desserts and, to a lesser degree, in savory dishes.

hors d'oeuvre   French for "outside of work" (the "work" being the main meal), an hors d'oeuvre can be any dish served as a starter before a meal.

horseradish   A sharp, spicy root that forms the flavor base in many condiments from cocktail sauce to sharp mustards. Prepared horseradish contains vinegar and oil, among other ingredients. Use pure horseradish much more sparingly than the prepared version, or try cutting it with sour cream.

hummus   A thick, Middle Eastern spread made of puréed garbanzo beans, lemon juice, olive oil, garlic, and often tahini (sesame seed paste).

insulin   A hormone secreted by the pancreas responsible for helping tissues utilize glucose and amino acids.

Italian seasoning   A blend of dried herbs, including basil, oregano, rosemary, and thyme.

julienne   A French word meaning "to slice into very thin strips."

kalamata olives   Traditionally from Greece, these medium-small, long black olives have a smoky, rich flavor.

ketosis   A process that occurs when the body goes through a prolonged period of starvation that produces dangerously high levels of ketones. Or, when the body ingests large quantities of fat in the absence of carbohydrates producing a minimal increase of ketones. In this case, ketones substitute for glucose as an energy source.

magnesium   An essential nutrient required for all energy-producing reactions that take place in the cells and muscles, including the ability to relax.

marinate   To soak meat, seafood, or other foods in a seasoned sauce, called a marinade, which is high in acid content. The acids break down the muscle of the meat, making it tender and adding flavor.

marjoram   A sweet herb, a cousin of and similar to oregano, popular in Greek, Spanish, and Italian dishes.

matchsticks   A reference to the shape of ingredients prepared by julienning. The food should be cut into long, thin strips.

meld   To allow flavors to blend and spread over time. Melding is often why recipes call for overnight refrigeration and is also why some dishes taste better as leftovers.

mince   To cut into very fine pieces smaller than diced pieces, about ⅛ inch or less.

mold   A decorative, shaped pan in which contents, such as mousse or gelatin, set up and take the shape of the pan. A mold can be made of metal, plastic, or silicone.

nonessential amino acids   Protein builders produced by the body utilizing raw materials supplied by food.

nutmeg   A sweet, fragrant, musky spice used primarily in baking.

olive oil   A fragrant liquid produced by crushing or pressing olives. Extra-virgin olive oil—the most flavorful and highest quality—is produced from the first pressing of a batch of olives; oil is also produced from later pressings.

olives   The fruit of the olive tree commonly grown on all sides of the Mediterranean. Black olives are also called ripe olives. Green olives are immature, although they are also widely eaten. *See also* kalamata olives.

oregano   A fragrant, slightly astringent herb used in Greek, Spanish, and Italian dishes.

oxidation   The browning of fruit flesh that happens over time and with exposure to air. Minimize oxidation by rubbing the cut surfaces with something acidic such as a lemon half. Oxidation also affects wine, which is why the taste changes over time after a bottle is opened.

paprika   A rich, red, warm, earthy spice that also lends a rich red color to many dishes.

Parmesan   A hard, dry, flavorful cheese primarily used grated or shredded as a seasoning for Italian-style dishes.

parsley   A fresh-tasting, green leafy herb, often used as a garnish.

pecans   Rich, buttery nuts native to North America that have a high unsaturated fat content.

peppercorns   Large, round, dried berries ground to produce pepper.

pinch An unscientific measurement term, the amount of an ingredient—typically a dry, granular substance such as an herb or seasoning—you can hold between your finger and thumb.

pine nuts (also **pignoli** or **piñon**) Nuts grown on pine trees, that are rich (read: high fat), flavorful, and a bit pine-y. Pine nuts are a traditional component of pesto and add a wonderful gentle crunch to many other recipes.

portobello mushrooms A mature and larger form of the smaller crimini mushroom, portobellos are brown, chewy, and flavorful. Often served as whole caps, grilled, and as thin sautéed slices.

preheat To turn on an oven, broiler, or other cooking appliance in advance of cooking so the temperature is at the desired level when the assembled dish is ready for cooking.

purée To reduce a food to a thick, creamy texture, usually using a blender or food processor.

reduce To boil or simmer a broth or sauce to remove some of the water content, resulting in more concentrated flavor and color and a thicker texture.

reserve To hold a specified ingredient for another use later in the recipe.

rice vinegar Vinegar produced from fermented rice or rice wine, popular in Asian-style dishes. Different from rice wine vinegar.

ricotta A fresh Italian cheese smoother than cottage cheese with a slightly sweet flavor.

roast To cook something uncovered in an oven, usually without additional liquid.

rosemary A pungent, sweet herb used with chicken, pork, fish, beef, and especially lamb. A little of it goes a long way.

roux A mixture of butter or another fat and flour, used to thicken sauces and soups.

salsa A style of mixing fresh vegetables and/or fresh fruit in a coarse chop. Salsa can be spicy or not, and served as a starter on its own (with chips, for example) or as a condiment with a main course.

sauté To pan-cook over medium or high heat using a small amount of oil.

sesame oil An oil, made from pressing sesame seeds, that's mild if clear (made from raw seeds), and aromatic and flavorful if brown (made from toasted seeds).

shellfish   A broad range of seafood, including clams, mussels, oysters, crabs, shrimp, and lobsters. Some people are allergic to shellfish, so take care with its inclusion in recipes.

shiitake mushrooms   Dark brown mushrooms with thin caps and a hearty, meaty flavor. Can be used either fresh or dried, grilled or as a component in other recipes, and as a flavoring source for broth.

shred   To cut into many long, thin slices.

simmer   To boil gently so the liquid barely bubbles.

skillet (also **frying pan**)   A generally heavy, flat-bottomed metal pan with a handle designed to cook food over heat on a stovetop or campfire.

skim   To remove fat or other material from the top of liquid.

slice   To cut into thin pieces.

smoke point   The temperature at which a cooking oil begins to smolder, causing it to break down and leaving it unfit to eat.

sodium   An essential nutrient that is required for the normal functioning of muscle and nerve cells. Excess amounts of sodium can lead to water retention.

steam   To suspend a food over boiling water and allow the heat of the steam (water vapor) to cook the food. A quick-cooking method, steaming preserves the flavor and texture of a food.

stew   To slowly cook pieces of food submerged in a liquid. Also, a dish that has been prepared by this method.

stock   A flavorful broth made by cooking meats and/or vegetables with seasonings until the liquid absorbs these flavors. This liquid is then strained and the solids discarded. Can be eaten alone or used as a base for soups, stews, etc.

superfood   A food that provides health benefits above and beyond basic macronutrients. These foods may help lower our risk of developing disease such as heart disease, type 2 diabetes, and cancer.

thyme   A minty, zesty herb.

toast   To heat something, usually bread, so it's browned and crisp.

tofu   A cheeselike substance made from soybeans and soy milk.

vegetable steamer   An insert for a large saucepan or a special pot with tiny holes in the bottom designed to fit on another pot. The holes allow steam from boiling water in the pan underneath to pass through and steam food held in the pot. *See also* steam.

vinegar   An acidic liquid widely used as dressing and seasoning, often made from fermented grapes, apples, or rice. *See also* cider vinegar; rice vinegar; white vinegar; wine vinegar.

walnuts   A rich, slightly woody flavored nut.

whisk   To rapidly mix, introducing air to the mixture. Also, a cooking utensil consisting of interlocking loops for this purpose.

white mushrooms   Also known as button mushrooms. When fresh, they have an earthy smell and an appealing "soft crunch."

white vinegar   The most common type of vinegar, produced from grain.

wine vinegar   Vinegar produced from red or white wine.

wok   A traditionally round-bottomed pan with a deep, sloping side for quick-cooking.

yeast   Tiny fungi used in dough. When yeast is introduced to heat and moisture, it releases carbon dioxide bubbles, which cause the bread to rise.

zest   Small slivers of peel, usually from a citrus fruit such as a lemon, lime, or orange.

zester   A kitchen tool used to scrape zest off a fruit. A small grater also works well.

The Quick Flour-Free Guide

With your newfound knowledge of flour-free cooking, you have the opportunity to venture out on your own. This appendix provides more information about utilizing flour alternatives as a replacement for wheat flour. Because these flour alternatives don't contain gluten, you'll need to add a binder, such as xanthan gum, in order to give your baked good the proper structure. In each recipe, you add 1 teaspoon of xanthan gum for every cup of flour alternative.

To utilize these flour alternatives, you need to know how they are substituted for wheat flour. Following is a list of these alternatives and the percentage replacement for flour in a recipe. Alternatives that are 100 percent replacement work as a one-to-one substitution for wheat flour. Those alternatives that are 25 percent replacement need to be combined with other alternatives in order to fully replace the flour in a given recipe.

- **Almond meal**—In substituting for wheat flour, almond meal can replace up to 100 percent of the flour in the recipe. Because of its increased density, use ½ cup of almond flour for every 1 cup of wheat flour.

- **Amaranth**—In substituting for wheat flour, amaranth can replace up to 25 percent of the flour in the recipe.

- **Brown rice meal**—In substituting for wheat flour, brown rice meal can replace up to 50 percent of the flour in the recipe.

- **Flaxseed meal**—In substituting for wheat flour, flaxseed meal can replace up to 100 percent of the flour in the recipe.

- **Ground chia seeds**—In substituting for wheat flour, ground chia seeds can replace up to 25 percent of the flour in the recipe.

- **Ground coconut**—In substituting for wheat flour, ground coconut can replace up to 20 percent of the wheat flour. For every ¼ cup of ground coconut, an equivalent ¼ cup of water (because of ground coconut's high fiber content) should be added to the recipe. The exception to this is in cakes and cookies, where ground coconut can replace up to 50 percent of the flour in a recipe.

- **Ground fava beans**—In substituting for wheat flour, ground fava beans can replace up to 25 percent of the flour in the recipe.

- **Ground garbanzo beans**—In substituting for wheat flour, ground garbanzo beans can replace up to 25 percent of the flour in the recipe.

- **Ground hazelnuts**—In substituting for wheat flour, ground hazelnuts can replace up to 33 percent of the flour in the recipe.

- **Konjac noodles**—In substituting for wheat flour, konjac noodles can replace up to 100 percent of the flour in the form of pasta or as a thickener in the recipe. As a thickener, 1 teaspoon of konjac is equal to 10 teaspoons of corn starch.

- **Quinoa**—In substituting for wheat flour, quinoa can replace up to 50 percent of the flour in the recipe.

- **Sorghum**—In substituting for wheat flour, sorghum can replace up to 20 percent of the flour in the recipe.

- **Steel-cut oats**—In substituting for wheat flour, steel-cut oats can replace up to 100 percent of the flour in the recipe.

- **Stone-ground cornmeal**—In substituting for wheat flour, stone-ground cornmeal can replace up to 100 percent of the flour in the recipe.

The following table gives you potential flour-free combinations for creating your favorite baked goods. For example, one recipe for cookies requires 80 percent steel-cut oats and 20 percent quinoa. This means that every 1 cup of flour is replaced by ⅘ cup of steel-cut oats and ⅕ cup of quinoa.

Suggested Alternative Flour Combinations for Flour-Free Cooking

Recipe	Flour-Free Combination
Bread	a. 50% flaxseed meal
	25% amaranth
	25% sorghum
	b. 35% flaxseed meal
	35% quinoa
	30% brown rice meal
	c. 33% ground garbanzo bean or fava bean
	33% brown rice meal
	33% flaxseed meal
Brownies	a. 50% amaranth
	25% ground coconut
	25% sorghum
Cake	a. 50% amaranth
	50% ground coconut
	b. 50% stone-ground cornmeal
	50% almond meal
	c. 33% ground hazelnuts
	66% almond meal
Cookies	a. 80% steel-cut oats
	20% quinoa
	b. 50% almond meal
	50% steel-cut oats
	c. 20% ground chia seeds
	40% brown rice flour
	40% almond meal

continues

Suggested Alternative Flour Combinations for Flour-Free Cooking   (continued)

Recipe	Flour-Free Combination
Cupcakes	a. 33% almond meal 33% amaranth 33% ground coconut
Muffins	a. 40% flaxseed meal 40% amaranth 20% quinoa
	b. 50% flaxseed meal 35% almond meal 15% brown rice meal
	c. 60% brown rice meal 20% steel-cut oats 20% flaxseed meal
Pancakes or waffles	a. 100% stone ground cornmeal
	b. 75% almond meal 25% sorghum
	c. 50% almond meal 50% brown rice meal
Pie crust	a. 60% quinoa 40% almond meal
	b. 50% steel-cut oats 25% ground chia seed 25% almond meal
Tortillas	a. 66% stone-ground cornmeal 33% brown rice meal

The following table provides some alternative choices for some more popular foods.

Alternative	Popular Uses
Almond meal	Pie crust, cookies, and as a sauce thickener
Amaranth	Breads, noodles, pancakes, cereals, and cookies
Brown rice meal	Breads, cookies, and muffins
Flaxseed meal	Muffins, cakes, cookies, and pie crust
Ground chia seeds	Muffins, cakes, cookies, and pie crust
Ground coconut	Breads, cakes, pies, desserts, cookies, pancakes, and waffles
Ground fava beans	Breads, pizza, cakes, and cookies
Ground garbanzo beans	Breads and crackers
Ground hazelnuts	Muffins, cakes, and cookies
Konjac noodles	Pasta substitute
Quinoa	Breads and as a rice substitute
Sorghum	Breads and porridge
Steel-cut oats	Breads, muffins, and cereals
Stone-ground cornmeal	Hot breakfast cereal, breads, pancakes, and muffins

Resources

To learn more about flour alternatives and where to buy them, look to these websites. Several websites about healthful eating are also included.

Almond Board of California
www.almondsarein.com
Here you'll find more information about almond meal, as well as tips and recipes.

Alvarado Street Bakery
www.alvaradostreetbakery.com
A source for sprouted-grain breads with web ordering and a store locator.

Asia Rice Foundation
www.asiarice.org
Learn more about brown rice and view helpful tips and recipes.

Barry Farm Foods
www.barryfarm.com
An online store for all your ground flour alternative needs.

Beans for Health Alliance
www.beansforhealth.com
An excellent resource for information on garbanzo beans as well as other dry beans, including nutritional information and recipes.

CarbSmart

www.carbsmart.com

A source for low-carb, sugar-free, and diabetic-friendly products with great customer service.

Chia Seeds

www.eatchia.com

A source for all you need to know about chia seeds.

Coconut Info

www.coconut-info.com

Check here for information regarding the use of ground coconut, including health information and suggested recipes.

Department of Health and Human Services (HHS)

www.health.gov/dietaryguidelines

Your electronic source for access to the Dietary Guidelines for Americans, due to be updated in 2010.

Fava Beans

www.fava-beans.com

Visit this website to learn more about fava beans, including nutritional information and recipes.

Flax Council of Canada

www.flaxcouncil.ca

All you need to know about flax can be found on this website.

Food for Life

www.foodforlife.com

Find information on sprouted-grain breads and cereals along with a store locator.

Hazelnut Council

www.hazelnutcouncil.org

Check here for more information about hazelnuts, including health benefits, nutritional information, and suggested recipes.

Konjac Foods

www.konjacfoods.com

Learn more about how to cook with konjac noodles.

Lakeside Mills

www.lakesidemills.com

This website has a lot of excellent suggested recipes utilizing stone-ground cornmeal.

McCann's Irish Oatmeal
www.mccanns.ie
Learn all you need to know about using steel-cut oats.

My Pyramid
www.mypyramid.gov
Use the personalized eating plans and interactive tools to manage your diet.

National Honey Board
www.honey.com
Find information and recipes for honey here.

National Metabolic Society
www.nmsociety.org
Visit this website to learn more about the impact of blood glucose and insulin. Also, you can view the latest research on diabetes and obesity.

Northern Quinoa Corporation
www.quinoa.com
Check out this site for recipes, tips, and health information on quinoa.

Nu-World Foods
www.nuworldamaranth.com
If you're looking for suggestions regarding amaranth, this is your web destination.

Nutrition Data
www.nutritiondata.com
This site provides the nutritional breakdown of all your favorite foods and food ingredients.

Nutrition.gov
www.nutrition.gov
Access U.S. government information about food and nutrition here.

Trader Joe's
www.traderjoes.com
Sellers of sprouted-grain breads, pasta alternatives, and other healthful food options with an online store locator.

Twin Valley Mills
www.twinvalleymills.com
Log on here for information about sorghum, including health benefits, suggested uses, and recipes.

Index

M

U–V

W–X–Y–Z